Steppping Stones to Electro-Homoeopathy

(Count Mattie's System of Medicine)

A.J.L. Gliddon

Second Editon-Considerably Enlarged

Originals
Delhi-110052

First Published 1892
Second Enlarged Edition with New Introduction 2017

Aurelius James Louis GLIDDON

ISBN 13: 978-81-8454-171-7
ISBN 10: 81-8454-171-6

Published By
Originals
A-6, Second Floor, Nimri Commercial Centre,
Ashok Vihar Phase-4, Delhi - 110 052 (India)
Tel.: +91 11 2730 2453 Fax: 011 4706 1936
website: www.Lppindia.com
e-mail: info@Lppindia.com

Printed At
D K Fine Art Press P Ltd.
Delhi-110052

PRINTED IN INDIA

Introduction

Stepping Stones to Electro Homoeopathy (Count Mattei's system of medicine,) was written at the request of the Count by A.J.L. Gliddon, enriched by his experiences and provided with his portraits, Electro Homoeopathy deals more with an electric "fluid" which is called bio-electricity of plants. It includes a catalogue of diseases cured by electro-homeopathy with the indication of the remedies of curing them. It has been published from Central Mattei Depot, London in 1893. It is by means of a theory the simple, with curative agents which he called Electricity in the remedies (Electro-Homoeopathy), so elementary that everyone may cure himself and his medicine is certainly the medicine of the future.

Stepping Stones to Electro Homoeopathy is by means of a theory of the simple yet effective therapeutic school, with curative agents which he termed Electricity in the remedies (Electro-Homoeopathy), so elementary that everyone may cure himself and Electro Homoeopathy medicine is certainly the medicine of the future.

Prof. Dr. Debasish Kundu Ph.D.

Prof. Dr. Debasish Kundu Ph.D.

M.D.H., F.F.Hom, F.I.H.M.S., Ph.D.(U.S.A.), D.Sc.(Colombo)

Fellow of International Holistic Medical Society, CA, U.S.A.

Fellow of Foundation of Homeopathy, NY, U.S.A.

Fellow of World E.Homeopathy System of Medical Council, Hong Kong,

Faculty, International Holistic Medical Society, CA, U.S.A.,

Vice-President, American Nutritional Medical Association, CA,U.S.A.

Visiting Professor, Khulna Homeopathic Medical College & Hospital, Khulna, Bangladesh.

Former Director General, Mooreland University, U.S.A.

Author:

Materia Medica for the New Age Man,
Diseases of Women,
Natural Medicines,
A Clinical Treatise on Cancer,Aids & Homeopathy,
Pharmacodynamics,
Aids & Your Sex Life,
Aids & Homeopathy,
Essentials of Acupuncture, etc.

Recipient, Royal Assyrian Order of Merit

Laureate, Dag Hammarskjold Award for Medicine

Editor In Chief, International Journal of Homeopathy & Natural Medicines, Science PG, USA

Editor in Chief, The Internet Journal of Herbal and Plant Medicine, U.S.A.

CONTENTS.

ERRATA.

Page 10—For Canal read *Canals.*
" 32—For Electro-homœpathy read *Electro-Homœopathy.*
" 34—For Cephalgia read *Cephalalgia.*
" 34—Line 6—For combatting read *combating.*
" 35—Line 15—For exosostis read *exostosis.*
" 37—Line 5—For ricketty read *rickety.*
" 42—Line 10—For Hemiphlegia read *Hemiplegia.*
" 42—Line 27—For inflammed read *inflamed.*
" 45—Lines 16 and 28—For prostrate read *prostate.*
" 46—Line 10—For Anascara read *Anasarca.*
" 49—Line 6—For prostratic read *prostatic.*
" 52—Line 17—For prostrate read *prostate.*
" 57—Par. 3—For tip read *sips* and for finger read *fingers*
" 69—Oils. After "hot water" add *or half drachm of Electricity*; and after "sweet oil" add *of almonds.*
" 93—Last line—For choral read *chloral.*
" 108—For Plegmasia read *Phlegmasia.*
" 138—For Cephalagia read *Cephalgia.*
" 139—For billious read *bilious.*
" 150—For Derryshire read *Derbyshire.*
" 203—Before "cancer of" read *Liver.* (The following three paragraphs refer to the liver).
" 209—For Menieère's read *Menière's.*
" 242—For Aphthœ read *Aphthæ.*

HOW TO PREPARE THE DILUTIONS AND EXTERNAL APPLICATIONS.

First Dilution (1).—Dissolve one first dilution globule (*i.e.* one of the little pills, not, as some suppose, a whole tube-full of them) in a six-ounce bottle or three-quarters of a tumblerful of distilled water, or water which has been boiled.

The globule may readily be broken up with a spoon after it has been allowed to stand in water for a few minutes.

Litre Dilution (L).—Dissolve one first dilution globule in four teaspoonfuls of water, and put one teaspoonful of this into a tumblerful of water, or dissolve one globule in a French wine bottleful of water, *i.e.*, in $1\frac{3}{8}$ pint.

Second and third dilution globules have been prepared (marked second dilution or third dilution) from which the second and third dilutions respectively can be prepared exactly as the first dilution is made from a first dilution globule.

Those who have only first dilution globules may prepare the second dilution thus:

Put one teaspoonful of the first dilution into a second six-ounce bottle and add water so as to fill up the whole bottle or three-quarters of the tumbler.

The Third Dilution may be prepared from the second dilution, thus: Put one teaspoonful of the second dilution into a third six- ounce bottle and add water as in the second dilution. It is generally advisable to commence treatment with the intermediate or second dilution.

Patients who suffer from heart disease, hysteria or epilepsy, generally require the third dilution.

WHEN FIRST DILUTION GLOBULES ARE USED NO GLOBULES ARE TO BE PUT INTO THE SECOND OR THIRD GLASS BOTTLE.

When the second or third dilutions alone are needed, it will be convenient to form the first dilution by dissolving one first dilution globule in a one-ounce bottleful of distilled or boiled water. Ten drops of this medicated fluid put into a six-ounce bottle or three-quarters of a tumblerful of water will form the second dilution.

The dilutions may be kept for use as long as the water remains good. The addition of a little spirit will serve to keep them pure. The glasses containing them should always be covered. BE SURE TO SHAKE OR STIR UP the dilutions before using them.

OMISSIONS.

DEAFNESS, *Congestive: Blue* El. to back and base of ear (keep the mouth open while the application is being made to the latter place), *Ang. 3* ointment to same places. *Ang. 1* second dil.

Nervous: Red or *White* El. to back and base of ear.

HIP DISEASE: *Scrof. 1* second dil. alt. *Canc. 4* second dil., *Red* El. to 14, 8. *Canc. 5* ointment.

PILES, *Blind: Scrof. 1* lit. dil. *Canc. 5* ointment. Sitz-baths of *Canc. 5* alt. *Ang. 3.*

Bleeding: Ang. 3 or *2* second or third dil. *Blue* El. and *Ang. 3* ointment to seat of affection. Sitz-baths of *Ang. 3.*

NOTE.

The figures referring to nerve centres, contained in the directions given from page 105 to page 251, refer to the points indicated on pages 102, 103, which are not in all cases identical with those in the diagram. In the next edition this want of harmony will be corrected, as it is likely to cause confusion.

PREFACE.

THE Author has had the privilege of interviewing and corresponding with a large number of persons who have wished to become acquainted with the best methods of using Count Mattei's medicines. He has thus learnt both what the majority of students of the new medical system most wish to know, and also what they find it most difficult to ascertain from the handbooks which have already been published. He has discovered that there is a real need of just the kind of book which he has striven to produce. In the following pages he has endeavoured to provide heads of families, clergymen and others with sufficient information respecting common diseases, and the best methods of treating them to render it possible for them to make good use of the interval between the discovery of disease and the appearance of a medical adviser, or to treat simple complaints when the assistance of a medical man is not deemed necessary.

This book has been written chiefly for the benefit of those who have already become convinced of the value of the Mattei medicines. It is, however, also designed to supply inquirers with such information and evidence as may serve to lead these to try them.

The introductory chapters contain answers to some of the objections which have been raised against the remedies. And the appendix supplies a brief epitome of the treatment which has proved successful in combating various serious diseases, including some which are usually regarded as incurable.

Count Mattei has suggested a few simple tests which may serve to convince inquirers that his remedies possess the properties which he attributes to them. Every one will have an opportunity of performing one or two of these interesting experiments. The old adage says that the proof of the pudding is in the eating. It is equally true that the proof of the medicine is in the using. Those, therefore, who doubt the statements made by Matteists with reference to the Count's mysterious drugs had better test them for themselves and see whether the following things do not occur.

(1.) A compress of Green Electricity will relieve articular pains, the pains of external Cancers and pains from any kind of ulcer.

(2.) 10 to 20 Globules of Scrofolso, will sober an intoxicated person, provided he is not an habitual drunkard.

(3.) 1 to 3 Globules of the same remedy, together with the application of Red Electricity to the pit of the stomach, will cure an attack of nervous indigestion.

(4.) Compresses of Blue Electricity applied to a bleeding wound, will stop hæmorrhage, relieve pain and promote cicatrization.

(5.) A few drops of Bluè Electricity poured into the palm of the hand and applied lightly over the heart, will relieve palpitation.

The Author is greatly indebted to Miss R. of Hampton Wick and to Dr. C. Stirling Saunder, of 64, Welbeck Street, Cavendish Square, for many valuable hints and for assistance in correcting the proofs. He will feel obliged to any other careful observers who will report to him the results of their experiments with the various Mattei Remedies, and will welcome any suggestions which are likely to assist him in preparing a revised edition of the present work.

A. J. L. GLIDDON.

Sarnia,
Melrose Road,
Wandsworth. S. W.

DIAGRAM OF HUMAN BODY to facilitate the EXTERNAL APPLICATION of ELECTRO-HOMŒOPATHIC REME

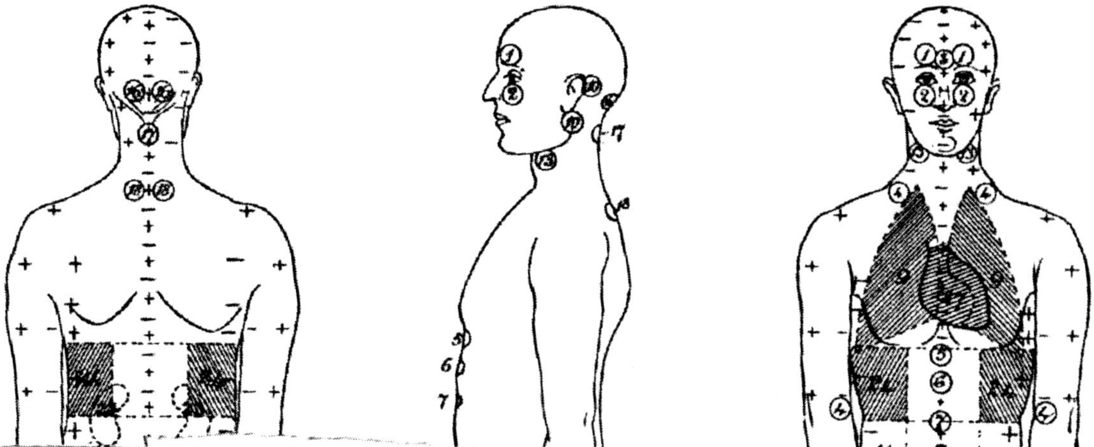

BLADDER: 20, 22, 25, 18
EARS: 10, the auditory canal, under the ear, the hollow at angle of jaw (when the mouth is opened)
EYES: 1, 2, 3 and temples
HEAD: 3, 16, crown of head, back of head and temples
HEART: Put 2 or 3 drops on palm of hand and pass gently

LEG: 8, 14 and sole of foot,
NOSE: 3, 1, 2
SEXUAL ORGANS: 20, 22, 25, 18
TONGUE: 16
WOMB: 20, 22, 25, 18

Drawn by C. Stirling Saunder, L.R.C.P. Lond

STEPPING STONES
TO
ELECTRO-HOMŒOPATHY.

INTRODUCTION.

HEALTH is the condition which results from the harmonious performance of the various functions of the bodily organs. Disease is the state which follows the rupture of this harmony. It ordinarily involves more or less pain and discomfort, and is generally dreaded in proportion as it is painful. It is the aim of medicine to prevent the commencement of discord, to restore harmony when it is lost, or, at least, to remove as much as possible of the pain and discomfort which usually accompany disease. Thus medicine is said to be preventive, curative or palliative.

The importance of preventive medicine is being increasingly recognised. It is found to be far better to use a prophylactic, as the preventive remedy is called, to check the advent of a malady than to wage war with it after it has acquired possession of the human frame. And thus it happens that many who believe themselves to be in special danger of being attacked by consumption, cancer, or even sea-sickness, are ready to welcome preventive medicines.

But it is still towards the curative and palliative remedies that men's chief attention is turned. Everywhere there are sufferers crying out for healing remedies. Few, indeed, are able to say that they have no need of these. Some who feel the need believe that no earthly power can supply it. But, even when they have no hope of finding a medicine which can cure their ailment, they anxiously seek for one which can relieve it.

The history of medicine is a history of perpetual experiments. The most diversified tactics have been adopted by the combatants with disease. Some of these have been of the most singular character. Charms and spells have been relied on as well as various substances derived from the animal, vegetable and mineral kingdoms. The lancet has been inserted to draw off blood and it is now sometimes employed to open the way for the introduction of blood. Electric appliances, baths, compresses, massage have been resorted to. And even the aid of light, colour, sound, heat and cold, have been sought. Some have held that drugs should have no place in the treatment of disease, while others have maintained that to neglect these is to display ingratitude for one of the chief gifts of the Creator.

Among modern users of drugs there are some who maintain that all remedies should be derived from vegetable substances, and others who seek for them also in the animal or mineral kingdoms. The latter class includes the orthodox school of medicine as well as the majority of homoeopathy. That which differentiates allopaths from homoeopathy is not a difference of opinion about the drugs which are useful for curing illnesses, but rather about the laws which should regulate the application of these drugs. The allopaths cannot be said to have a law. For, although they are popularly believed to oppose the homœopathic plan of administering for the relief of a disease the very drug whose action upon a healthy organism produces an effect most like the symptoms of that affection, they do not carry out their opposition consistently. Again and again they are found practising in harmony with the law which they profess to defy. But it is not so with the homœopaths. These strongly maintain that "like cures like," and choose all medicines under the guidance of this great principal. They hold that the human organism is a sworn foe to disease, and that no sooner does discord commence than it seeks to quell it. When left alone it frequently succeeds in curing itself. And when artificial aid is imparted it seems natural that this aid should be so administered as to help the organic forces to work more rapidly and more powerfully on the lines along which they would work if left to themselves. Since, then, the homœopath simply pushes a moving train in the same direction in which it is already moving, it is evident that he need not introduce much additional force in order to produce a striking effect. The use of a small dose is, therefore, exactly what might be expected. The weight of a pin may be all the additional pressure which is requisite to enable nature to bear down some great obstruction. The traditional straw which breaks the camel's back does this because it is the last integer added to a whole series of weights which are pressing in the same direction. There is in Cornwall an enormous rocking or balancing stone which a few years ago was pushed down a cliff by a mischief-making tourist. It is easy to imagine that this stone might have been in such a state of unstable equilibrium that a child's push would have sufficed to thrust it down the cliff. It would have sufficed to do this, not because the child's power was in itself capable of moving that mass through that space, but because the forces of nature were already at work, and were tending to pull the stone downwards. The push would have done wonders because it worked with nature. But while the child's push would have sufficed to move the stone downwards, how vastly different a degree of force would have been requisite to pull it upwards again. This simple illustration may suffice to show that the minute dose of the homœopath is neither unphilosophical nor absurd.

As a result of careful study and deep and prolonged thought on medical subjects Count Cæsar Mattei became a confirmed homœopath many years ago.

But when he had entered the homœophatic school he discovered that the medicines at the homœopath's disposal were quite insufficient. There were many diseases which he could not cure, and some for which he could afford but little relief. He, therefore, determined to seek for new remedies.

While in this state of mind he noticed that a favourite dog of his, who suffered from a skin affection, went, day after day, as he accompanied his master on his walks, to a particular plant, ate some of its leaves, and continued doing so until he was completely freed from this complaint. This discovery convinced Count Mattei that the dog's instinct had led him to the true medicine, and he forthwith determined to ascertain the extent of the medicinal value of the plant of which the dog had partaken. Being an amateur chemist he had no difficulty in extracting its active principle. When this was done he tried its effect upon certain sufferers with whom he was acquainted, and was delighted to find that the results of treatment surpassed his highest anticipations. A series of experiments convinced him that he had discovered a new drug of enormous worth, and one whose sphere of action was very wide. But he soon found that he could reach its limits. Persons of Angioitic or sanguine temperaments failed to derive that benefit from its use which had so markedly followed its presentation to lymphatic sufferers. Encouraged, however, by the great discovery which he had made in so curious a fashion the Count devoted himself very energetically to the study of the physiological action of the active principles of other plants, and was rewarded by discovering a remedy of singular value in the treatment of those diseases which are peculiar to persons of sanguine temperaments, and also several other precious medicines.

A series of experiments, conducted in various parts of the world during more than a quarter of a century, has shown that the medicines discovered by Count Mattei are among the most valuable remedies known to men. They have been found to possess the power of assisting the healing force of nature in its warfare with almost all kinds of disease. And they have displayed this power even in relation to some forms of illness which have hitherto been regarded as incurable. So marvellous have been the effects which have followed the wise use of these remedies that a growing company of disciples regard Count Mattei as the only medical teacher with whose drugs they need concern themselves. Other admirers of this medical discoverer are unwilling to abandon the older remedies which have been proved to be really valuable. But both classes are anxious to know what is the best that can be done by means of the Mattei medicines in the treatment of the principal diseases. For the sake of helping both, the following pages have been prepared. They give more fully and yet more succinctly than any previous publication what experience has shown to be the best hints for the treatment of each of the most familiar diseases, and of a number of rarer ailments.

I. THE HUMAN BODY.

AS this handbook is written chiefly for the sake of helping those who have had no medical training, to use the Mattei Remedies successfully, it has been thought advisable to include in it a brief physiological sketch.

The several parts of the human body have been classified by anatomists into eight systems : (1) the osseous system ; (2) the muscular system ; (3) the alimentary system ; (4) the circulatory system ; (5) the absorbtive system ; (6) the respiratory system ; (7) the excretory system ; and (8) the nervous system. To the first belong all the bones ; to the second all the muscles ; to the third the pharynx, œsophagus, stomach and intestines ; to the fourth the heart, arteries, capillaries, and veins ; to the fifth the absorbent vessels or lymphatics ; to the sixth the larynx or voice box, the trachea or wind pipe, and the lungs ; to the seventh the liver, the kidneys, the lower bowel, and the skin ; and to the eight the brain, spinal cord, nerves, and ganglia.

The central part of the skeleton is known as the *vertebral column* or back bone. The latter designation is inaccurate, as there is really a series of back bones, of which twenty-four are movable on each other, and nine are so united as to be incapable of separate motion. The seven uppermost vertebræ, or neck bones, are called *cervical* vertebræ from the Latin word cervix, the neck. Below these come twelve bones which are called the *dorsal* vertebræ, because they are the bones of the back (dorsum, the back). Lower still are the five bones of the loins called *lumbar* vertebræ (lumbus, the loin). Then come the first five closely fused vertebræ forming the *sacrum* (Lat. sacred). And last of all come the bones of the rudimentary tail, which are thought by many to point to the fact that our ancestors possessed tails. These four imperfectly formed vertebræ compose the *coccyx*.

The bones of the skull are divided into two groups (1) those belonging to the brain box or cranium and (2) the facial bones. The former include the sphenoid bone, shaped like a flying bat, and forming part of the base of the skull, the occipital bone forming its back and the other part of its base, two parietal bones forming its sides and roof, the frontal bone, the two temporal bones, or bones of the temples, and the spongy sieve-like ethmoid bone through which the branches of the nerves of smell pass to the nose from the brain. The bones of the face include the two nasal bones which form the bridge of the nose, the two turbinated bones, curved round like scrolls, projecting into the nasal cavities, and separated by a very thin bone called the vomer, the two lachrymal bones between the nose and the eyes, which contain the ducts through which tears pass from the eyes to the nose, the two molar or cheek bones, the two superior maxillary bones forming the upper jaw, and the inferior maxillary forming the lower jaw.

The bones of the upper limb include the clavicle or collar bone, the scapula or shoulder blade, the humerus or upper arm, the ulna and radius (the bones of the fore-arm) the eight carpal or wrist bones, the five metacarpal bones, which connect the fingers and thumb with the wrist, and the fourteen phalanges or finger bones. The bones of the lower limb are the two pelvic or hip bones, the femur or thigh bone, the patella or knee cap, the tibia or shin bone, the fibula or splint bone, the seven tarsal or ankle bones, the five metatarsal or instep bones, and the fourteen phalanges or toe bones.

The bones are bound together by means of strong white fibrous bands or ligaments, and are connected with muscles by means of other white bands or tendons. They are produced by a hardening process from cartilage or gristle. This hardening process during the early years converts only a part of the cartilage of the infant into bone. The other portion remains as a permanent cartilage. But in aged persons some of this becomes hardened by the absorption of lime. Thus it happens that the vertebral columns of the aged become stiffened.

Some joints, such as those of the skull, are movable and others are immovable. The former include gliding joints, ball and socket joints, hinge joints, and pivot joints. The articulating surfaces of these are covered with cartilage, and this is covered with the synovial membrane, from which exudes a fluid known as the synovial fluid, by means of which the joints are lubricated.

The parts of bones which are not situated at joints are covered with a tough fibrous membrane known as the periosteum. Small vessels pass from this into the bone and unite with the Haversian canal whose diameter averages $\frac{1}{800}$ of an inch. From this minute canals radiate in all directions into what are known as the lacunæ. Through this series of extremely minute vessels the circulation of the blood is carried on within the bones.

The muscles are divided into the voluntary muscles, which are under the control of the will, and the involuntary muscles, which are not subject to the authority, of the will. Both of these are composed of bundles of fibres, whose diameter averages about $\frac{1}{500}$ of an inch, and which are formed of still smaller bundles of fibres. These have the power of contraction and produce motion by means of this contraction. This contraction may be caused by irritation, whether this be mechanical, chemical, or electrical. Every fibre of a voluntary muscle is enclosed in a thin tough sheath, which is known as sarcolemma.

The body contains two chief cavities, the great cavity and the cavity of the skull and spinal cord. The former is divided into the thorax or chest and the abdomen, or belly, by means of a muscular partition known as the diaphragm or midriff. The alimentary canal passes through this cavity. There are other minor cavities. Of these the uppermost is the nasal cavity. The air passes into this from without through the nostrils and thence through the two posterior nares into the pharynx.

Another smaller cavity—the mouth—also communicates with the pharynx. The fleshy substance forming its roof extends backwards beyond the hard palate and forms the soft palate. Behind this is the pharynx, which communicates with the middle ear by the eustachian tubes and which is continued downwards to the œsophagus, or gullet, as the passage is called, which leads from it into the stomach. From the pharynx a tube called the trachea or windpipe extends into the lungs. The upper part of this, which forms what is known as Adam's apple, is the larynx or voice-box This contains the bands of elastic fibres by whose vibration the voice is produced. The opening between the pharynx and the larynx is called the glottis. Attached to this is a lid (the epiglottis) which opens during breathing and speaking but closes while the act of swallowing is being performed, and so prevents the food from passing into the windpipe.

The windpipe passes into the chest or thorax and divides the upper part of this into two tubes known as the bronchi, one of which enters each lung. Like two great branches of a tree these tubes divide and subdivide. The very minute twig-like air tubes penetrate every part of the lungs. At their extremities are groups of air-cells which have extremely thin walls.

The lungs are spongy bag-like organs, penetrated with arteries which divide and subdivide like the branches of the bronchi, until at their extremities we find exceedingly small vessels ($\frac{1}{3000}$ of an inch in diameter) called the capillaries. These capillaries form a net work and surround the walls of the air-cells. The oxygen of the air breathed into the bronchial tubes passes through the walls of the air cells into the capillaries. And here a highly important exchange takes place. The carbonic acid which has been collected from all parts of the body, and brought by the blood corpuscles through the arteries into the lungs, is passed out through the walls of the air-cells and exchanged for the oxygen which has been drawn into the air-cells by means of the act of inspiration or breathing. The blood thus freed from its impurities, and enriched by this oxygen, passes into other capillaries, and thence through the pulmonary veins into the heart. The lungs are surrounded by a membrane called the pleura, another layer of which lines the chest walls.

The heart occupies the middle portion of the front of the chest. It contains four cavities, the right auricle, the right ventricle, the left auricle, and the left ventricle. Between the two former is the tricuspid valve. Between the two latter is the bicuspid or mitral valve. The other valves of the heart are the two sets of semilunar valves, situated respectively at the junction with the heart of the pulmonary arteries and the aorta. The heart is surrounded by membrane known as the pericardium which, like the pleura, is composed of two layers. In this case, however, the second layer serves as a loose envelope.

It has already been stated that the œsophagus leads from the mouth to the stomach. It passes behind the windpipe, between the lungs, and then through the diaphragm, immediately below which it widens out into the stomach. The latter is a pear-shaped pouch at whose other end is the pylorus, an opening into the small intestine, which is about twenty feet in length. This unites with the large intestine, which is about six feet in length, at a point where there is situated the cæcum or blind intestine, which is a kind of pouch. The part of the large intestine between the cœcum and the rectum is called the colon. Flatulence is often felt in its ascending, transverse, or descending section.

Just below the stomach is situated the liver, which is the largest gland in the body and forms about $\frac{1}{40}$th of its entire weight. It consists of two lobes. Each of these lobes is made up of small lobules about $\frac{1}{20}$th of an inch in diameter. Between the blood vessels with which the liver is well supplied there are minute liver cells about $\frac{1}{1000}$ of an inch in diameter, by means of which the blood is deprived of bile which is passed into the gall bladder, to be poured thence into the duodenum, where it aids in digesting food. Sometimes, however, it passes directly into the duodenum.

Behind the stomach is the sweetbread, or pancreas, which also secretes a fluid for digestive purposes. Close to the pancreas is the spleen or melt, a ductless gland, whose function is not well understood, although it is believed by many to be engaged in the manufacture of the red corpuscles.

Beneath all these are the kidneys, which are situated on each side of the backbone, and which are covered with fibrous coats called capsules. The kidneys separate from the blood a watery fluid which contains much of its nitrogenous waste matter. This is conveyed through the ureter into the bladder, whence it is periodically discharged.

The bladder is situated behind the pubis. In women the womb occupies a place at the rear of the bladder. The ovaries are found on each side of it, between it and the groin.

Around the abdominal organs there is a membrane called the peritoneum, whose outer layer lines the inner surface of the abdomen. Certain of its folds, which join parts of the intestines with the posterior walls of the abdomen, are called the mesenteries.

Throughout every part of the complex organism which forms our earthly tabernacle there is a wonderful system of nerves. This is divided into two parts. The more important of these is called the cerebro-spinal system and consists of the brain, the spinal cord, and the nerves which spring from them, and are extended into the organs of sense and the voluntary muscles. The other part of the nervous system is known as the sympathetic system, and consists of two chains of knots and of a few disconnected knots of nervous matter or ganglia. One of these chains is situated on each side of the spine. The fibres which originate in this system penetrate the internal organs and the walls of the blood vessels.

The nerve centres, such as the brain and spinal cord, are largely composed of a grey substance. The nerves themselves are really bundles of fibres, of which some are white and others are grey. Some of the nerves are said to be sensory or afferent nerves, because they bring to the centres what we know as sensation, such as that of pain. Others are called motor or efferent nerves because they carry from the centres those impulses which cause muscular fibres to contract, and so produce motion in various parts of the body.

II. COUNT MATTEI'S THEORIES.

CRITICS must not suppose that if they can show the falsity and folly of Count Mattei's theories they can thus deal a death-blow to the reputation of his remedies. Nor must non-critical readers, who find it difficult to accept or perhaps even to understand the theories, imagine that this need deter them from using the remedies. The remedies are not so closely linked to the theories that they must stand or fall together. Count Mattei has no hesitation in confessing that while the efficacy of his remedies is readily demonstrable, it is not so easy to prove the correctness of his theories. Notwithstanding this, it will interest our readers to know something of the latter.

In order, however, that they may be understood certain truths must be learnt and remembered. A brief epitome of these will be serviceable to some.

It is well-known that the human body is dependent for its continued life upon the soil and atmosphere. It is no mere poetic figure which represents man as dust of the ground vitalised by the air or breath which God has produced. But in order that the body may retain its vitality and undergo development, it is necessary that the elements which the earth supplies for his use should undergo several great changes. The first of these is effected by means of various forms of vegetation, which gather different substances from the soil and the atmosphere, transform the inorganic into the organic, and so prepare the former a becoming food for sentient organisms. A further change is effected by means of those of the lower animals which enter into the dietary of our race. And after vegetable or animal food has been introduced into the mouth of man it has to pass through a wonderful series of transformations ere it has fulfilled its high function of sustaining the lord of creation.

The food which has been introduced into the mouth there undergoes a double process of preparation for future use. By means of the teeth it is cut and ground down into smaller pieces, and is at the same time subjected to the influence of a colourless secretion which is poured into the mouth from the parotid, submaxillary and sublingual glands. This fluid not only separates the particles of food and prepares them for being acted upon by the other digestive fluids, but also lubricates it, and so makes the act of swallowing easier than it otherwise would be. Its most important work, however, is to effect a chemical change in the starchy elements of food. These it alters into sugary substances.

After undergoing this preliminary digestive process the food is transferred to the stomach. It is retained in this elongated pouch for a considerable time, and is here acted upon by a slightly viscid fluid, known as the gastric juice, which exerts a most potent influence over the nitrogenous articles of food. These it not only dissolves but converts into substances called peptones. A considerable part, however, of the albuminates are not completely peptonised, but are simply transformed into what Meissner called parapeptones. The peptones are supposed to be at once absorbed by the mucous membrane. The remaining semi-fluid mass, including fatty matters which are not digested in the stomach, is passed intothe small intestine where it undergoes a further process of digestion. Two important fluids are here poured upon the food. The first of these is the bile. This apparently acts as a natural purgative by stimulating the action of the intestinal walls, and also promotes the absorption of fatty matters. The second is the pancreatic juice, a strongly alkaline colourless fluid. Its action resembles that of the saliva, than which however it is much more powerful. Other juices take part in intestinal digestion. One is poured out of a set of minute tubes which are found in the mucous membrane of the small intestine. It is known as intestinal juice. After being acted upon by this, a further portion of the food is taken up into the circulation by means of some extremely minute projecting bodies, called villi, about $\frac{1}{30}$ of an inch in length. These are provided with capillaries, through which a portion of the fluids in the intestines is absorbed directly into the blood. But a larger portion is taken up through lacteals which are found in the interior of these villi. The unabsorbed portion of the food as it passes on further is subjected to the action of fluids secreted by Brunner's glands, Peyer's glands, and some solitary glands which are found in all parts of the intestine. It is not known what is the precise work done by each of these. The insoluble residue is expelled from the body.

The lacteals, by which, as we have just seen, some of the changed food (or chyle) is absorbed, form part of the lymphatic or absorbent system. The minute vessels containing the lymph are found in nearly every texture and organ of the body, and are arranged in a superficial and a deep set. The latter are larger than the former. The structure of the lymphatics resembles that of the veins and arteries. At certain places such as the neck, the axilla, the groin, the abdomen, and the chest, there are small bodies known as lymphatic glands. Not only do the lymphatics, as we have seen, collect new materials for the formation of blood, but they also serve as channels through which effete matter is carried off from the tissues into the veins.

Because the chyle is of a milky colour and gives to the vessels which absorb it a milky appearance, these are called lacteals or white vessels.

The white lymph as it passes through the mesenteric glands becomes more highly organised. It is then carried forward until it reaches the spot where it is poured into the blood.

That part of the chyle which is preserved for the uses of the organism consists of water, albumen, sugar, fat, and mineral salts. Under the influence of the pancreatic and intestinal juices and the bile the sugar is changed into fat. The nutritious extract may then be regarded as an aqueous solution of albumen, fatty bodies, and mineral salts.

Albumen is the chief ingredient in the white of an egg. It also exists in the sap of vegetables. Its chief constituents are carbon (which forms 54 °/o of it), hydrogen, nitrogen, and oxygen, with small proportions of phosphorus and sulphur.

The food has now been transformed into impure or VENOUS BLOOD. This is poured into the right auricle of the heart which contracts and drives it through the tricuspid valve into the right ventricle. This in its turn contracts and sends the venous blood forward into the pulmonary artery, from which it is distributed through the minute capillaries which are found in all parts of the air-cells contained in the lungs. Here the impure blood comes into direct contact with the oxygen of the air which the man inspires, and as it combines with this and becomes oxidised it is rendered capable of becoming, as Mattei puts it, "the plasma of tissues and the potential element of phenomena which jointly constitute the manifestation of the organic life of a being."

By means of a series of oxidations the various parts of the body are built up or repaired from the materials contained in the blood. Thus is formed the syntonin of which the muscles are made, and which is composed of carbon, hydrogen, nitrogen, oxygen, and sulphur. Thus, too, are made the sides of the blood vessels, the connecting sub-cutaneous tissues, and the whole mass of matter which, on boiling separates in the form of a jelly. The fat which gives the body its suppleness and elasticity is drawn from the blood current. So, too, are the mineral elements which form the frame of the solid parts. "Nothing except the form is contained in the tissues which did not pre-exist in the blood."

The channels along which the nutritive fluid is borne to all parts of the system are at first comparatively large.

But from these large channels there branch out other and smaller channels from which, as from the branches of a tree, other stems are put forth. This process is continued until at the extremities of the channels we find an extremely delicate and complicated network, known as the capillary system. The average diameter of the capillaries in the muscular tissue is 0·003 of a line. In the brain their average is still less. Some of these little vessels are so small that only one blood corpuscle can pass through them at once.

The nutritive fluid is carried through these channels at a gradually decreasing rate. Under the influence of chemical attraction and affinity it parts with certain of its elements to the neighbouring tissues. It is, according to Mattei, a general law of the organism that "the different elements which traverse it are separated from the fluid which carries them," when they reach places where they are specially needed. The living molecules in the organic woof which is penetrated by the blood sort out, by a species of elective affinity, the materials which they need to replace effete or corrupt elements.

If, through some defect in the blood or lymph, an element which no longer plays a useful part in a tissue continues there it deranges life and so causes disease. The same thing happens if it is expelled and no element replaces it. The restoration to the organism of its natural mode of action can only be effected by the expulsion of the effete element and the substitution of an element which is *similar* to what the effete element was in its normal condition. Only a similar element can fill the place which is or must be vacated, and do the needed work. To introduce such an element is to administer a medicine. And only that can be considered a true medicine which will thus re-establish the natural functions.

This is what Mattei means when he says "Life is in the blood, disease in its vitiations, and medicine in similars." This is what he means when he implies that disease is also in the vitiations of the lymph and that medicine in this case, too, is in similars.

According to his view the human organisation is entirely built up by, and so dependent upon, the lymph and the blood. If these two liquids are in a perfectly normal state the whole body will be healthful. As the old and worn-out or super-oxydised elements are eliminated from the system by perspiration through the skin, by expiration through the lungs, or by excretion by means of the kidneys, &c., and carried back to the inorganic world whence they came, the blood and the lymph will supply similar new elements to take their places. And by this admirable process of decomposition and recomposition life and health are continued. If, however, either the lymph or the blood, or both, are so vitiated that they cannot supply the tissues with the matter which they require in place of that which has become super-oxidised, disease ensues.

To remedy this vitiation Mattei believes it to be necessary to use remedies which can correct the abnormal symptoms manifested in different parts of the organism. If true remedies be discovered, and exhibited to the organism in a subtle and dynamized form, he holds that the lymph and the blood will take up into themselves the elements needed to effect their cure. These will at once have a medicinal influence. The true curative medicine, therefore, must be a reconstructive food.

It has been found by experiment that the remedies of the Antiscrofoloso group of remedies are capable of curing diseases which result from the vitiation of the lymph. And it is therefore believed that the remedies in this group supply the lymph with the elements which are needed by the parts to which it bears the nutritive fluid. And when it is found that any particular disease is curable by the Antiscrofoloso group of remedies it is concluded that it results from the vitiation of the lymph.

Similarly it has been proved by repeated experiment that medicines of the Antiangioitico group are capable of curing diseases which result from the vitiation of the blood. And it is consequently thought that the remedies belonging to this class introduce into the blood those elements which are required by the tissues and vessels to which it carries the necessary food. When it is discovered that any particular disease is curable by the Antiangioitico series of remedies it is concluded that this disease is consequent upon the vitiation of the blood.

A third series of experiments has shown that certain other diseases resulting from the vitiation both of the blood and of the lymph which are incurable by the Antiscrofoloso group alone, or the Antiangioitico series only, can be healed by means of a combination of the two. When it is found that any disease needs both classes of remedies, it is thought that it results from the vitiation both of the blood and of the lymph. Hence Mattei has laid down the axiom that diseases which require the same remedy, or the same remedies, have a common origin, that is to say they originate in a vitiation of the blood, of the lymph, or of both.

The remedies which he exhibits have the power of bringing back the constituent elements of all parts of the body to their normal condition in cases where they are administered in time. And as Nature banishes her own foes when she herself is strong, the Matteist, by purifying her life current, gives her the victory over at least some of her enemies.

While the remedies supply the organism with the elements it needs, they help it to drive away those for which it has no use. Hence under their influence foreign and morbid principles are expelled from the frame by abundant perspirations, by expectorations, by urinary deposits, by boils or by diarrhœa.

Patients who use the right remedies must, therefore, not be surprised if these symptoms manifest themselves. Of course they must not be allowed to become excessive. Should this happen a higher dilution of the medicines must be used.

III. SYMPTOMS OF DISEASE.

THE existence of disease in the body is proved by the presence of certain abnormal conditions, which are known as the signs or symptoms of disease. To ascertain by means of an examination of these symptoms what is the nature of the disease which has taken possession of the body is, in the language of medicine, to diagnose the disease. It is impossible in the course of a brief chapter to state all the physical and other signs by means of which the presence of particular diseases may be ascertained. But it will be useful to give a few of these in a concise form.

1. **Pain.**—This is generally the symptom which induces the patient to seek a cure. In many cases he is quite content if he can remove this, even though the disease which has originated it should not be expelled from his body. Pain resides in the nervous system and may result from its abnormal stimulation on the one hand, or its unnatural relaxation on the other. There are various kinds of pain, *e.g.*, dull, gnawing, tearing, burning pains, &c. In some diseases it is continuous. In others it is intermittent. It may exist in the diseased organ or tissue, or in some other part of the body. It is

well to remember that pain in the left arm may be caused by heart disease, pain in the head by indigestion, pain in the right shoulder by inflammation of the liver or diaphragm, pain at the outlet of the urethra by stone in bladder, pain in the knee by hip disease. Severe pains at the back of the head are often found in Bright's disease. Pain as of a nail being driven into the head accompanies Chlorosis. Deep-seated crushing pains occurring regularly at night are indications of the presence of syphilitic virus.

2. **Disordered Circulation.**—The heart may beat too fast or too slow, It may beat irregularly. It may palpitate. When its action is excessive it produces a congested state of the blood vessels, with consequent sense of rushing of blood to the head, dull headache, giddiness, noises in the ears, specks before the eyes, enlarged veins, hæmorrhage and a tendency to dropsy and skin diseases, such as erythema, eczema, &c. When its action is deficient there is a tendency to faintness, coldness of the extremities, &c. The normal sounds of the heart may be replaced by others as a result of defects in the valves, &c.

3. **Colour.**—By carefully observing the colour of the patient's skin, and especially of his face, a medical man is often greatly helped in diagnosis. Certain diseases of the heart or lungs produce a dusky or livid hue, while others produce a bluish tint. In Bright's disease the patient's face presents a blanched, pasty and puffy aspect. In biliary affections there is a yellowish colour in the face. Anæmic girls are pale and waxy looking, while in those

who suffer from chlorosis, a greenish or yellowish-green hue may be observed. Most of those who are suffering from cancer sooner or later become straw-coloured. A rich circumscribed blush points to irritability of the nerves or disease of the lungs.

4. **Breathing** should be closely observed, especially if there is any suspicion of disease of the lungs or bronchi. In phthisis respiration is usually abnormally rapid and becomes more so towards evening. Abnormal frequency also characterises anæmia, hysteria, fevers, and some kinds of cardiac affections. In bronchitis there is a sense of oppression, weight or tightness in the chest. In trance and apoplexy the breathing is often abnormally slow. Dyspnæa, or difficult breathing, characterizes some organic and functional diseases of the heart, effusions into the pleura or pericardium, asthma, &c.

5. **Temperature.**—The average temperature of the healthy body taken at the axilla is 98·4. It undergoes a daily rise and fall of from 1·8° to 2·3° Fahr., being lowest at from 2 a.m. to 6 a.m. and rising until from 5 p.m. to 8 p.m. It may sink to 97·3 or rise to 99·5 or even to 100. But if it passes beyond these limits it may be taken for granted that there is some disease at work in the system. We cannot too strongly urge heads of families to keep a clinical thermometer in their homes, and to get into the habit of taking the temperature of any one of the members of the household who may fall ill. The presence of a serious disease may thus be revealed when only a slight ailment has been suspected. In

measles the pyrexia is moderate at first, about 100°, and rises continuously up to the height of the rash, when the temperature is not usually above 103°. In scarlatina there is high pyrexia at first, about 100, which rises to 104°, 106° or even 108°. In small-pox the temperature rises rapidly to 104° or 106°, falls speedily when the eruption appears, and then rises again to 104° or 105°. In typhus fever the temperature rises regularly up to the fourth or fifth evening, when it reaches 104° or even higher, falls slightly on the sixth morning, but rises again in the evening. On the seventh morning there is a marked fall followed by another rise. In typhoid fever there is a regular rise of 2° each evening followed by a regular fall of 1° each morning. The height reached at night is ultimately 104° to 106°. In intermittent fever the temperature rises several hours before the paroxysm sets in. In consumption the temperature is raised to 102·3° or even higher. In rheumatic fever the temperature ranges from 100° to 104°, and there is generally a considerable difference between the morning and evening temperatures. Sometimes it rises to 109°, 110°, 112°, and may even continues to rise after death for a short time.

6. **State of the Tongue.**—Few doctors fail to ask their patients to show them their tongues. And no wonder. For, even with reference to disease, the tongue is a great tell-tale. A livid or purple tongue declares that the blood is imperfectly oxygenated. A tongue which is covered with a yellow coat announces that the liver is disordered. A furred tongue speaks of irritation of the mucous membrane, and is generally present in almost all

acute illnesses. In enteric and typhus fevers the tongue is deeply fissured, and in scarlatina its surface resembles that of a strawberry. In gastric and bilious fevers, and in serious attacks of dyspepsia, the tongue is abnormally red.

7. **The Expression** often materially assists the practitioner in forming his diagnosis. Mania, epilepsy, hysteria, &c., have their characteristic expressions.

8. **The Condition of the Excretions** needs to be specially noted.

(i.) The urine should not only be examined whenever there is any suspicion of disease in the urinary organs, but also in many other cases, for its condition gives important information respecting other maladies. In nervous ailments it is pale. In gout and rheumatic fever it is abnormally acid. In jaundice it has a saffron colour. In fever it is red or high coloured. In some affections of the kidneys or bladder it is bloody or slimy. In acute Bright's disease it is dark, its specific gravity rises to 1025, 1030, 1040 or more, its odour resembles that of beef-tea, and an abundent brown and flocculent sediment forms. In chronic Bright's disease it is of light colour and low specific gravity. In diabetes it is increased in quantity. The act of voiding it often causes pain or irritation, and is more frequently performed than is healthy. It is generally sweetish to taste and smell, ferments rapidly, is very clear and pale, has a high specific gravity (over 1030), and contains from 8 to 12 per cent. of sugar.

(ii.) The fæces. Discharges of unaltered food point to arrest of the digestive functions. Watery evacuations are symptomatic of intestinal irritation. The presence of bile in stools is indicative of congestion of the liver.

9. **Cough** is symptomatic of various diseases. Any direct or reflex irritation of the larynx, trachea, or bronchial tubes may give rise to it. Thus it may be caused by the presence of worms, by teething, by an unhealthy condition of the heart, the liver, the ear, or the female generative organs.

10. **Spitting of Blood.**—This accompanies various diseases of the larynx, trachea, bronchi, lungs or heart; such as cancer, phthisis, congestion of the lungs, mitral disease, hypertrophy of the left ventricle.

11. **Dropsy.**—This may arise from heart disease, acute bronchitis complicating extensive emphysema, disease of the kidneys or liver, the pressure of a pregnant uterus, ovarian and other tumours, aneurisms, varicose veins of long standing, impoverishment of the blood, or the irritation of cancer.

12. **Eruptions** must be noted. Certain forms of these point to acute and others to chronic specific diseases. In measles the eruption generally appears on the fourth day, and is first seen on the forehead or other part of the face. It consists at first of minute red points, which grow into papules. These tend to form patches of crescentic shape. In scarlatina the eruption appears the second

day, on the neck. There are minute points at first, which coalesce to form patches, or to cover the whole surface of the body. In typhoid fever the eruption consists of a few rose-coloured spots situated on the abdomen, chest and back, which are slightly raised and disappear on pressure. In typhus the eruption is first seen about the back of the wrists and on the axillæ and epigastrium. It consists of dusky red mottling and mulberry-coloured spots. The eruption in small pox is first seen on the face. It consists of small bright red spots which form into hard shot-like pimples. These become in succession vesicles, pustules, and scabs.

IV. THE ELECTRO-HOMŒOPATHIC REMEDIES.

MANY people have enquired why Count Mattei has given the name "Electro-Homœopathic" to his remedies. It has already been shown that the remedies act homœopathically. And this has revealed the reason for the latter part of the compound name. But why use its first part?

The narrative of the discovery largely answers this question. In the course of his experiments with several liquids which he had prepared, Count Mattei found that certain morbid affections disappeared by simply touching the seat of disease with these liquids, and that these acted with electric speed and produced an electric effect. He was perfectly astonished, and concluded that he had discovered new forms of vegetable electricity. He still clings firmly to this idea, although he has since called the liquids electroids or electric remedies, and has given his followers the alternative of supposing that the true explanation of their effect may be that the nervous system is in an electrotonic state, and that on the contact of the liquid with the skin, at the points where the nerves are nearest the surface, there is developed by it an electro-motor force.

It has been scientifically demonstrated that muscles

and nerves exercise a very regular and comparatively powerful electric action. Even the skin is itself somewhat electrically active. The bottle-shaped or skin glands have been shown to possess regular electric activity. The base of each of these glands is positively electric, while the upper surface is negatively electric. Rosenthal maintains that "every nerve, every muscle and every part of a muscle when quiescent is positive on its longitudinal section; negative on its cross section." It may be that the fluids stimulate the electric activity of the nerves. But, as we have stated, Mattei strongly favours the view that electricity is contained in the fluids, just as truly as other forms of it are contained in batteries and leyden jars.

As the vegetable essences which are used in preparing the globules, as well as those which are found in the fluid remedies, are believed to embody this force, Count Mattei has called his remedies "Electro-Homœopathic."

It is important to bear in mind that while homœopathy and allopathy are generally content to combat symptoms, Electro-homœpathy directly attacks the causes of disease. Finding these primarily in the vitiation of the lymph and the blood, and in the consequent disorganisation of the vessels containing them, it sets to work to restore these fluids and their channels to their normal condition. It does not, however, altogether ignore the symptoms or neglect the relief of pain, &c., during the period which must elapse ere the foundations of the evil shall have been destroyed.

THE GLOBULE REMEDIES.

Antiscrofoloso₁ or Scrofoloso 1.

The first place in the series of remedies is occupied by *Anti-Scrofoloso 1.* This medicine is formed of the active principles of one or more plants, whose names have not been allowed to transpire. It was at first regarded by its discoverer as a panacea. But, after a while, he found that it did not produce such good effects in persons of sanguine as in those of lymphatic temperament. Nevertheless, he still maintains that as, according to Hahnemann's proofs, herpes, psora, or scrofula is to be found in a more or less attenuated form in every constitution, all treatments may begin with this remedy. For it has the power of ridding the system of the germs with which it is generally impregnated, and which tend to debilitate and destroy it. By doing this it prevents the appearance of many diseases which otherwise would ravage the body. And, as prevention is better than cure, it forms an invaluable assistant to those who cherish health. So instantaneous is its action that a few globules of it will restore a person who has fainted, arrest an attack of indigestion, if given at the commencement, and even restore an intoxicated person, provided he be not a habitual drunkard. Two or three granules of the same remedy taken dry on the tongue will give appetite, stop cramp in the stomach, relieve toothache, (especially if this is associated, as it so often is, with digestive disorders) and produce sleep. The aged will find it very useful in preserving energy and elasticity. It has also the power of removing unpleasant symptoms caused by an overdose of any of the other Electro-homœopathic remedies. It is useful in scrofulous and rachitic affections, glandular enlargements, the disorders resulting from the abuse of mercury, sciatica, paralysis, "grippe" (*i.e.*, Influenza), and chilblains. It is, like Venereo, anti-syphilitic, and should be used in combatting latent or hereditary syphilis, with or without *Canceroso 1.*

It is best adapted to persons of lymphathic temperaments and to those of any other temperament who are subject to glandular enlargements and phlegmonous inflammations.

The following are some of the diseases for which it is generally useful, especially in the persons of the temperament for which the remedy is best adapted. Those of sanguine or mixed temperaments generally need some other or additional remedy. In cases which are complicated with bilious tendencies *Scrof. 5* is preferable to *Scrof. 1.* Albuminuria, Amaurosis (incipient), Amenorrhœa, Amygdalitis (chronic, resulting from herpetic diathesis), Anæmia (in second dil. with *Ang. 1* second dil.) in all disorders dependent upon it, Angina (catarrhal), Aphonia, Apthæ, Appetite (loss of), Apoplexy (nervous), Arthritis, Ascites (with general dropsy), Asthma (nervous, in scrofulous persons, excited by too great efforts or too large meals), Bladder (paralysis of the), Blenorrhagia, Blenorrhœa, Blepharitis, Boils, Bones (caries of the, tumours of the), Brain (concussion of the, inflammation of the), Breath (fœtid), Bright's Disease, Breasts (excoriation of the), Bronchitis, Bulimy, Carbuncles, Caries, Cataract (incipient with *Ang.* and *Mar.*), Cephalgia, Cephalo-Meningitis, Chills (a few globules morning and evening),

Chlorosis, Cholera (Asiatic or sporadic), Chorea, Cold in the head (first dil.), Colic, Constipation (obstinate, in lymphatic patients), Consumption of the Bowels, Convulsions, Cornea (spots on the), Coryza (chronic), Cough (nervous), Coxalgia, Cramp in the legs, nape of neck, stomach, also menstrual and ovarian, Cystitis, Deafness (nervous), Debility, Dentition (difficult), Diabetes, Diarrhœa (with or without vomiting: alternate with *Feb.* if this fail, or with *Canc. 1* if the stools are greenish-white), Diphtheria, Dislocation (spontaneous, in infants), Drowning (asphyxia from), Drunkenness (inclination to), Dyspepsia (when not bilious), Ear (disorders of the), Earache, Eczema (externally with *Scrof. 5* internally), Eclampsia, Elephantiasis, Enteritis, Epilepsy, Eruptions (chronic), Eruptions (retrocession of, through chill), Erysipelas (with *Ang.* or *Feb.*), Exhaustion, Exosostis, Eye (disorders of the), Fainting, Fevers (eruptive, with *Feb. 1*), Fevers (miliary, mucous, nervous), Fevers (sequelæ of), Fistulas (dental, lachrymal), Ganglions, Gastralgia (flatulent), Gastric ailments of pregnant women, Gastritis, Generative debility, Generative system (disorders of the), Glandular swellings, Glossitis, Gout, Gravel, Grippe with *Feb.*, Gums (affections of the), Hæmorrhoids (blind), Headache (sick), Hernia, Herpes, Hunger (morbid), Hysteria (in very weak doses of the third dilution), Idiocy, Impetigo, Impotence, Incontinence of urine, Indigestion, Insomnia, Intoxication, Itch, Kidney Diseases, Knee (swelling of), Lachrymal fistula (with a little *Canc. 5*), Laryngitis, Laughter (convulsive), Lepra, Lethargy, Lumbago, Lupus, Luxation of femur (spontaneous), Mania, Marasmus, Masturbation, Megrim, Melancholy, Meningitis (acute),

Mental disorders in men (for women use generally *Canc. 1*), Metritis (puerperal), Milk crust, Miserere, Myelitis, Nausea (even during pregnancy), Nephritis, Nerves (affection of the), Nervous agitation, Neuralgia in the head or stomach (non-congestive), Nose (disorders of the : Inflammation, Polypus, Swelling, Ulcerations), Nymphomania, Obesity, Odontalgia, Œdema of the pupil of the eye, Œsophagitis, Onanism, Ophthalmia (catarrhal, granular, syphilitic), Orchitis (through blows), Ottorhœa, Ovaries (acute inflammation of the), Ozœna, Paralysis (commencement of), Periostitis, Phlegmonous nose in scrofulous infants, Phthisis (intestinal), Piles (blind), Pleurisy, Pleurodynia, Pneumonia, Poisoning (effects of), Pollutions (nocturnal), Polypus of larynx and nose, Psoriasis, Pyrosis, Rheumatism (articular), Rickets, Scabies, Scarlatina, Sciatica (with *Feb.*), Scurf, Scurvy, Sea-sickness, Skin diseases (all kinds, in minute doses), Small-pox with *Feb* , Smell (loss of), Somnambulism, Sores (difficult to cicatrize), Spasms, Spermatorrhœa, Spina Ventosa, Spine (inflammation of the), Stammering, Staphyloma, Stone, Strangury, Stricture of the Urethra, Styes (tendency to), St. Vitus' Dance, Suffocation, Sweating of the armpits and feet, Syncope, Tabes mesenterica, Taste (loss of), Teeth (caries of), Teething (difficult), Tendons (retraction of the), Tetanus, Thrush, Thunder (effects of), Tongue (inflammation of the, paralysis of the), Tonsils (chronic inflammation of the), Toothache, Trismus, Tumours (while forming), Twitchings (convulsive), Ulcers, Urethritis, Urinary system (disorders of the), Urine (retention of the), Uterus (relaxation of, ligaments of), Vaccination (evil effects of), Voice (loss of), Vomiting (even of pregnancy), Wasting diseases in children, Wax in ear (hardened), Whitlow, Wounds which are inclined to cicatrize.

Scrofoloso 2.

Adapted, like *Scrof. 1*, to persons of lymphatic temperament. Useful in affections of Scrofulous and ricketty persons. Its action is deeper, but less extensive than that of *Scrof. 1.* It has the advantage of not exciting the vascular system as *Scrof. 1* sometimes does, and should be preferred to the latter when this causes constipation or light-headedness. It holds a position between *Scrof. 1* and *Ang. 1*, and may be used subsequently to *Scrof. 1*, to continue treatment.

It is specially useful in the treatment of Bladder (catarrh of), Blepharitis, Bulimy, Calculus (biliary), Catarrhal cough, Cephalagia (hystericand nervous), Chorea, Croup, Dyspepsia (nervous and chlorotic), Elephantiasis, Excoriation of the nipples, Gastric fever, Glandular swellings in the neck, Goitre, Gonorrhœa (chronic, with *Ven.*), Gout, Gravel, Hair (falling off, after acute illness), Hernia (infantile, through crying), Hydrocele, Itch, Leprosy, Migraine, Nervous excitement, Nettle rash (chronic), Neuralgia (hysterical), Nymphomania (after child-birth), Odontalgia (with swelling of jaw and sub-maxillary glands), Paralysis of hands, Pellagra, Rheumatic fever, with *Feb.*, Scabies, Sciatica, Scurf, Sores (non-cancerous), Suppression of milk, Taking cold, Ulcer of cornea, Warts, Wounds (to hasten cicatrization).

Scrofoloso 3.

Useful for outward application in Bruises, Burns,

Scratches, Wounds. May be taken internally for Angina of tonsils, Atrophy of scrofulous infants, Convulsions (infantile), Cramp (in calves of legs, menstrual), Debility (especially through seminal losses), Epilepsy (children), Gastralgia, Genital affections (through suppressed gonorrhœa), Genital weakness, Headache through abuse of alcohol or over study, Hernia, Herpes (facial, also of scrotum or pubes), Lockjaw, with *Yellow* El., Nodes (arthritic), Spermatic cord (inflammation of), Testicles (congestion of), Tongue (induration of).

Scrofoloso 5.

This splendid remedy occupies a position between *Scrof. 1* and *Canc. 1.* It has Anti-cancerous properties. Its sphere of action is very extensive and very deep. It produces brilliant effects in many digestive disorders, when, on account of chronic affections of the liver, *Scrof. 1* cannot be used, but should, in these cases, be associated with *Feb. 1.* It is especially useful in Skin diseases. It is used largely in baths, compresses, &c. Internally it is used for Angina (Granular), Boils, Calculus (renal), Carbuncle, Chilblains, Cold humours, Colic, Constipation (chronic), Coryza (chronic), Diarrhœa, Digestive disorders (especially those arising from retrocession of skin disease), Drunkenness (sequelæ of), Dysmenorrhœa (painful, in sterile women), Dyspepsia, ECZEMA, Elephantiasis, Glands (suppurating), Goitre, Gout, Gravel, Laryngitis (chronic, with ulceration), Lupus (nasal), Myelitis, Pains, Parotid with formation of abscesses or fistula, Phthisis (intestinal), Piles (blind), Rheumatism (chronic, aggravated during bad weather), Sciatica, *Skin disorders* (chronic),

Stings (insect), Stone, Typhoid Fever (with *Feb.*), Vomiting.

Scrofoloso 6

Is chiefly useful in Bladder Diseases, Bright's Disease, Indigestion through taking acid or cold beverages, Marasmus in adults, Melancholia, Muscular weakness with trembling of limbs, Pains after blows or falls, Rheumatic affections in joints of hands or feet, Scrofulous sores. Its action is said to be less extensive but deeper than that of *Scrof. 1.*

Scrofoloso Giappone.

This remedy is composed of *Scrofoloso* and *Febrifugo*, and is chiefly used in diseases where a frequently repeated and simultaneous action of *Scrofoloso* and *Febrifugo 1* is deemed necessary. Such are CHOLERA (in the treatment of which during the epidemic of 1883-4 *Scrof. Giap.* was marvellously successful), Cholerine, Diarrhœa, Dysentery, Fevers, (especially the more serious such as Typhus), Vomiting. It is useful as a preventive of Cancer, Grippe, Hay fever, and most Infectious Diseases; and also for the relief of most Digestive Disorders.

The Angioiticos.

These remedies act upon the heart and other parts of the vascular or circulatory system, and should be used both when these alone are disordered, and also when, as often happens, they are affected in consequence of some defect in the lymphatic system. In the latter case they must be alternated with one of the *Antiscrofolosos* or *Anticancerosos*. Whenever a disease of the liver is associated with a disease of the heart the *Febrifugos* must be alternated either with the *Angioiticos* alone, or also with the *Scrofolosos*.

The *Angioiticos* are useful to persons of sanguine temperaments in almost all their diseases. They are far superior to Aconite and Digitalis.

The following are the chief diseases which are treated by means of *Angioitico 1*, *2*, and *3*. Many of the diseases named in the following list under *Ang. 1* are now being successfully treated with *Ang. 3*, and the conviction is growing that it is generally better to commence the treatment of all *Angioitic* cases with the third in the series. No. 1 generally requires to be administered in such weak dilutions that No. 3 is now most generally used for internal treatment, except where a stronger action is required. It is also largely used for Baths, Ointments, and Compresses. If it is then found that a stronger remedy is needed, recourse may be had to *Ang. 1*. No. 2 is chiefly used externally.

In all cases when the pulse is rapid or the patient is peculiarly sensitive, and especially when the heart is diseased, it is well to commence treatment with the second or third dilution.

Antiangioitico, or Angioitico 1.

Anæmia (in Angioitic constitutions), Aneurism (a few teaspoonsfuls daily), Apoplexy (idiopathic or traumatic, with effusion of blood), Asthma (congestive), Blood (want of, with *Canc. 1*,) Boils, with *Scrof.*, Cerebral Congestion, Circulation (slow with *Canc. 1*,) Colic (menstrual), Congestion (in sanguine temperament), Cough (convulsive),

Cystitis, with *Scrof.*, Dysentery, Ecchymosis of eye, Encephalitis, with *Scrof.*, Epilepsy when arising from vitiated circulation, Epistaxis, Eyelids (inflamed, with *Scrof.* or *Canc.*), Eyes (spasms of the muscles of the), Fainting, Fevers (inflammatory) with *Feb.*, Generative organs (acute inflammation of), Gouty inflammations with swelling, with *Scrof.*, Hæmatemesis, Hæmaturia, Hæmoptysis, Hæmorrhage, Hæmorrhoids(fluent), Headache (congestive), Heart diseases (in cases of organic heart disease external treatment is of the first importance), Lethargy, Melæna, Meningitis (acute or chronic), Menstruation (too copious), *2nd* or *3rd* dil., Mental disorder (all sorts of), Metritis, Metorrhagia, Monomania, (acute attacks), Neuralgia, Paralysis (congestive), Piles (bleeding), Phlebitis, Pleurisy, with *Pet.*, Quinsy, Rheumatic affections (with swelling), Somnolence arising from congestion or inflammation of the brain, Sore-throat (acute and phlegmonous), Spitting of blood, Sunstroke, Syncope, Trismus (when symptomatic of cerebral inflammation), Typhoid fever, with *Feb.*, Varicocele, Vertigo, White swelling, Wounds.

Angioitico 2.

All disorders of the circulation in the arteries, heart and veins, Anæmia, Aneurism (externally in compresses), Angioitis, Aphthæ, Apoplexy (sanguine), Arterial hæmorrhage, Articular pains, Ascites (if from blood irritation), Asthma (with arterial hæmorrhage), Atrophy, Black eyes, Catarrh, with *Pett.*, Convulsions (during the menses), Cough (nervous), Congestion, Dropsy (cardiac, ovarian), Dumbness, Dysentery (with blood, first dil.), Dysmenorrhœa, Dysuria, with *Scrof.*, Ear disease (congestive), Ecchymosis of the eye, Encephalitis, with *Scrof. 3*, Enteritis, Elephantiasis, Epilepsy (when arising from defective circulation), Epistaxis, Erysipelas (phlegmonous), Eyes (hæmorrhage from the), Eyelids (spasms of the, with vertigo), Fauces (congestive pains of), Fistula of the Gum, with *Canc.*, Foot (swelling of), Gout, Gravel, Gums (disorders of the), Heart diseases, Hæmatemesis, Hæmaturia, Hæmoptysis, Hæmorrhage (from the eye, womb), Hæmorrhoids, Hemiphlegia (consequent on apoplexy), Hydrocephalus, Hydropericarditis, with *Canc. 2*, Hysteric disorders (arising from deficient vitality of the uterine system), Insanity (furious, third dil., with *Scrof. 3.*), Intercostal neuralgia (with suppression of the menses), Itch, with *Scrof.* or *Canc.*, Jaundice, with *Feb.*, Laryngitis, Leprosy, Leucorrhœa (obstinate cases), Lupus, Melæna, Metritis, Menorrhagia, Myelitis, with *Scrof.* or *Canc.*, Neuralgia (congestive), Nocturnal pollutions, with *Scrof. 2*, Obesity (morbid, with *Scrof.* or *Ven.*), Œdema, Otorrhœa, with *Scrof.* or *Canc.*, Ozœna, with *Scrof.* or *Canc.*, Paralysis (congestive), Patches, Pericarditis (third dil.), Pleurisy, Pneumonia with *Pet.*, Polypus of the womb, with *Canc. 2* or *4*, Prolapsus uteri, with *Canc.*, Proud flesh, with *Canc.*, Rectum (loss of blood from the), Rheumatism (articular), Rickets, with *Scrof.* or *Canc.*, Sciatica, Spitting of Blood), Throat (sore), Thrush, Ulcers (inflammed, scorbutic), Urine (incontinence of), Urine (retention of, in sanguine patients), Varices, Varicocele, Vertigo (from excessive blood), Wine-coloured spots on skin, Wounds (gangrenous) with *Canc. 4.*

Angioitico 3.

Abscess, warm (with *Canc. 1* during suppuration), Amygdalitis, Angina Pectoris, Apoplexy (hæmorrhagic), Arteries (diseases of), Aneurisms (dilatation, inflammation, hæmorrhage), Arteritis (congestive), Aorta (inflammation of the, thoracic, or abdominal), Asthma (congestive or vascular), Bladder diseases, Bronchitis (acute), Cancer, with *Canc.*, Carditis, Chilblains, with *Scrof. 1* or *Canc. 1*, if there is suppuration, Chlorosis, with *Scrof. 1*, Consumption, with *Canc.* and *Pet.*, Deafness (congestive), Dropsy, Dysuria (congestive), Dysentery (with bloody stools), Endocarditis (acute and chronic), Enteritis, Fevers (acute, inflammatory, alt. with *Feb.*), Fungus hœmatodes, Gastritis, Headache (congestive), Hæmorrhage (from the mouth, nose, anus, urethra, womb or wound), Heart diseases (aneurism, atrophy, cardiac dropsy with *Canc.*, endocarditis, hypertrophy, palpitation, pericarditis, valvular diseases), Herpes, Hydrocele with *Ven.*, Hydrothorax, Hydropericarditis, Laryngitis (chronic), Lungs (congestion of), Morbus ceruleus, Nettle rash, Palpitation, Panaris, Paralysis, Pericarditis, Phlebitis (functional or traumatic), Pneumonia, (acute and chronic), Quinsy, Scrofula, Skin disease (chronic, with *Scrof. 5*), Steno-carditis, Stomach (ulceration of), Sunstroke, Ulceration of the stomach, Ulcers, Varicose disorders, Veins (diseases of the, cuts, dilation, phlebitis), Varices, Varicose ulcers, Vertigo, Vesicle tenesmus.

Canceroso.

The *Canceroso* remedies belong to the same category as the *Scrofolosos*, but have a more powerful action.

They are used in cases which resist the action of *Scrofolosos*, such as cold abscesses, scirrhus, and other cancerous tumours.

The Anticancerosos or *Cancerosos* are best known as the remedies for cancer. It must not, however, be imagined that this is their only use, or that in cases of cancer they are the only remedies required. When the constitution is seriously affected at least two or three medicines are generally needed.

To ensure success in the treatment of cancer, it is necessary to begin using the remedies while the disease is in its early stage. When once the vital organs are deeply affected, and the disease is making rapid progress, the chances of cure are very small. Still, in these cases, relief of pain and prolongation of life may be promised. And sometimes brilliant results have followed a very late beginning of the treatment.

It is important to remember that the first effect of *Canceroso* is sometimes to aggravate the disease; that the process of cure is sometimes very slow, and that occasional pauses may be expected. But, when once the dose adapted to the patient's constitution has been proved, he may expect that, even though the waves in the tide of health bound back repeatedly, it is after all a flowing and not an ebbing tide.

The following are the chief diseases in which *Canceroso 1* may be advantageously used: Abscess of mammary glands, Amenorrhœa, Angina (gangrenous), Ascites, Bladder (catarrh of the, polypus of the, softening of the), Bones (diseases of), Breasts (congestion of the), Bronchial catarrh, Cancer of the anus, breast, intestines, lips, liver, nose, skin, stomach, tongue, uterus, &c., Carbuncle, Caries of the teeth and bones, Cataract, Catarrh (uterine, pulmonary, chronic), Cerebral congestion with vertigo, Colic, Condylomata, Congestions (uterine), Cysts (ovarian), Cramp (uterine), Diabetes, Diphtheria, Displacement of the womb, Dorsal marasmus, Dropsy (some forms of), Dysmenorrhœa, Enteritis, Facial lupus, Fainting spells, Falling of the womb, Fistula (dental, ani, vaginal), Gangrene, Gastritis (acute and chronic), Generative system (disorders of the, in both sexes), Granular laryngitis, Glands (suppurating), Goitre, or with *Scrof.* 5, Gout in the great toe with heat and redness of the skin, Gouty tumours, Hard swelling of the upper lip, Hectic fever, Hypertrophy of the neck of the womb, Hysteric attacks, with *Ang.*, Induration of the womb, Inflammation of the gums, nipple, parotid gland, prostrate gland, rectum or testes, tongue, womb, lungs, Itch, Labour (painful or prolonged), Laryngitis (granular), Leucorrhoea (chronic), Liver (induration of, with *Feb.*), Lung (congestion of the), Lung (inflammation of the), Lung disease (all kinds of), Lupus (facial), Mania (especially in women), Mesenteric Disease, Metritis (serous, granular, mucous), Miscarriage, Morning Sickness, Nausea (in pregnancy), Nervous disorders in pregnant and nursing women, Numbness of the arm, Obesity, Orchitis, Osteitis, Ovaries (affection of the), Parotiditis, Peritonitis, Phthisical symptoms, Phthisis (intestinal), Polypus of the bladder or uterus, Pregnancy (disorders of), Prolapsus ani, Prostatis, Prostrate (atrophy of, hypertrophy of), Pulmonary Tubercles, Quinsy, Rectum (inflammation of the), Ringworm, Scurvy, Softening of the brain, Spasms (especially uterine), Small-pox, Spinal disease, Strictures, Syphilis (in ulcerations), Tabes dorsalis, Throat (ulcerative or granular), Tuberculosis of bones, Typhoid fever, with *Feb.*, Urine (incontinence, retention), Uterine disorders, Ulcers in the leg, Vaginitis (acute and chronic), Varioloid disease, Wasting diseases of children, Whites, White Swellings, Womb (all diseases of), Wounds.

Canceroso 2.

This has a gentler and deeper action than *Canc. 1.* It is specially useful in Dropsy.

Amenorrhœa, Anascara, Anchylosis, Angina (scarlatinal), Angina (guttural, if obstinate), Arthritic affections, Ascites, Ascites with general dropsy dependent upon organic affection of the stomach, Bladder (catarrh of the), Brain (tubercles of), Breast (congestion of the), Cancer of the lips (scirrhus), Cancer of the womb, Carcinomative affections, Curvature of the spine, Dropsy, Dropsy of womb, or ovary, Epilepsy, Eyelids (spasms of the), Falling of the vagina and of the womb, Glandular inflammation, Gonorrhœa (bastard), Hepatitis, chronic, after the use of *Feb.*, Hepatitic phthisis, Hydrarthrosis, Hydrocele, Hydrocephalus (acute), Hydropericarditis, Hysteria, Laryngitis, Legs (Œdema, swelling of the), Leucorrhœa, Lips (scirrhus induration of the), Lung (chronic disorganisation of the), Loins (pain in, through a fall), Lymphatic vessels (inflammation of), Mastitis, Mesenteric disease, Miscarriage (premonitory symptoms and sequelæ), Melancholy (arising from uterine derangement), Nephritis, Œdema, Ophthalmia, Ozœna in scrofulous infants, Polypus of the womb, Puerperal peritonitis, Rheumatismal affections, Scarlatinal angina, Scirrhus affections, Spermatic cord (inflammation of), Spasms of uterus, Spinal curvature, St. Vitus' dance, Ulcers (inveterate), Ulcers (scorbutic), Wen in the head, Womb (cancer of the), Womb (pain in).

Canceroso 3.

Abdominal phthisis, Anchylosis, Arthritis (inveterate), Bubo (scrofulous), Cancer (in the lips, breast, heart), Cancerous ulcers, Carcinonatous ulcers, Catarrh (chronic), Coxalgia, Cysts, Dislocation, Exostosis, Inflammatory swelling of the knee, Necrosis, Paralysis of the joints of hands and feet either through rheumatic affection or dislocation, Periostitis, Pneumonia (chronic with suppuration), Ringworm, Spine (curvature of the), White swelling in the knee, Womb (ulceration of the).

Canceroso 4.

Abscess (congestive), Anchylosis, Angina (pseudo-membranous, second dil.), Bone diseases (inflammation, softening, suppuration of bone), Bone pains, when not resulting from syphilis, Cancer (pains of which do not yield to *Canc. 1*), Carbuncle, Caries of bones, Coxalgia, Cysts, Elephantiasis, Exostosis, Fistula of anus, Gangrene, Hip-joint disease, Humpback, Humours (cold), Hydrocele, Inflammation of the articulation, Lupus, Mumps, Myelitis, Necrosis of bones, Neuralgia (osteal), Nodes, Obesity, Ophthalmia, Osteomyelitis, Osteitis (acute and chronic), Panaris (bony), Periostitis, Periostosis, Phthisis, Piles (blind, some cases), Polypus of bladder, bowels, palate, nose, ear, womb), Prolapsus (rectum), Scald-head, Scrofula, Spina ventosa, Staphyloma, Syphilis, Tic, Tubercles of face (inflammatory), Tuberculous cough, Tubercular tumour of the belly, Ulcers (varicose, complicated with scrofula), Whitlow.

Canceroso 5.

The most powerful of all the *Cancerosos*. Very much used for baths, compresses, &c. Used also internally for:

Abscess, Acidity, Acne (syphilitic), Amaurosis, Anascara, Anchylosis, Angina (chronic tendency to), Angiotis, Amblyopia (amaurotic), Aphthæ, Asthma (spasmodic), Cancer in all external parts (lips, breast, eye, skin), also Cancer in womb, Capillary system (diseases of), Cataract, Chlorosis, Chorea, Convulsions (epileptic), Cramp (uterine), Deafness, Diarrhœa, Diphtheria, Dysmenorrhœa, Dyspepsia, Epilepsy, Eruptions (chronic), Eye diseases (chronic), Female ailments, especially in weak constitutions with delicate and sensitive skins, Fistula (lachrymal), Ganglionitis, Gastralgia and other Gastric affections, Glandular induration, or inflammation, Gonorrhœa (chronic, with *Ven.*), Hair (falling off), Heartburn, Herpes (chronic), Hysteria, Insanity, Labour pains (absence or excess of), Laryngitis, Laryngeal phthisis, Leucorrhœa, Lochia (too long duration of, suppression of), Mania, Megrim, Metritis, Miscarriage (tendency to), Nervous diseases, Nervous excitement with insomnia, Nocturnal pollutions, Paralysis, Phthisis, Polypus of womb, Pulmonary cavities, with *Pet. 2*, Ringworm, Scirrhus (induration), Scrofula, Scurvy, Stomach disorders (acute), Syphilis (in ulcers, &c.), Thrush, Typhoid fever, Ulcers (all kinds of), Wax (hardening of), Whites, Whitlow, Womb (cancer in, gangrenous affections of the).

Canceroso 6.

It has valuable tonic properties. Used in baths in cases of general weakness and cachexia.

Bilious disorders, with *Feb.*, Cancer in lips, Cholera (infantile), Cholerine, Cystitis, Diabetes, Diarrhœa (choleraic in infants), Ear discharges (purulent), Gastric disorders, with *Feb.*, Kidney diseases, Metrorrhagia (in weak and unhealthy women), Nephritis, Otorrhœa (purulent), Prostratic disease, Tumours (uterine), Typhoid fever, Urinary affections.

Canceroso 10.

Combines the action of the preceding numbers. Should only be used when the others fail, especially in—

Cancer formed on old cicatrices after actual abscesses, Cancer of the stomach, Cancer of the womb, Chancres (obstinate), Colic through strangulation of the intestines, Ozœna, Syphilitic herpes, Tabes dorsalis, Vomiting in pregnancy.

Canceroso T.B.

Should only be used under medical advice. Said to have been useful in the retention of urine.

Febrifugo 1.

The great remedy for diseases of the liver and spleen. Specific in all kinds of fever. It is also of great use in nervous disorders which spread from the nervous centres and the abdominal and thoracic ganglions of the sympathetic nerve, as well as in such conditions as ecstasy, somnambulism, spontaneous clairvoyance, consequent upon nervous disturbance of the solar plexus or semi-lunar ganglions.

Catalepsy, Cephalalgia (intermittent), Cholera, with *Scrof.*, Diabetes (some forms of), Diarrhœa, with *Scrof.*,

Digestive disorders, with *Scrof.*, Diplopia (when arising from a deep affection of the sympathetic nerves), Fainting (hysterical), Fevers (Intermittent, Periodic, Pernicious, Quartan, Quotidian, Tertian), Heart disease (nervous, with palpitation), Hepatitis (acute and chronic), Hepatalgia, Home-sickness, Hypochondriasis, Hysterical nervous attacks, Icterus or Jaundice, Kidney disorders, Liver, (congestion of, enlargement of, induration of, obstruction of), Nervous attack (resulting from various disorders), Neuralgic affections (periodic), Palpitation (nervous), Spasms of the larynx and throat (nervous), Spleen disorders (acute and chronic), Splenitis (acute and chronic).

Febrifugo 2.

Is always associated with *Feb. 1* in the diseases for which that remedy is required; it is applied in ointments and compresses to the hypochondria. Sometimes it is used internally in obstinate fevers (such as typhus) when they resist the action of *Feb. 1.* In this case it is given in the second or third dilution.

Pettorale 1.

Asthmatic pains, Bronchorrhœa, Bronchial irritation, Bronchitis (acute and chronic, capillary, follicular), Catarrhal cough, Cough (constant desire, caused by irritation or itching of the larynx), Cough (convulsive), Cough (nervous), Croup, Dentition (difficult), Feeling of weight and pressure on the chest in breathing, Laryngitis (rheumatic, acute, chronic, ulcerous), Lungs (chronic hepatization of the, chronic obstruction of the, œdema of the), Hooping cough, Pneumonia, Phthisis (pulmonary and tracheal), Pleurisy, Sore throat, worse in the afternoon and evening, Spitting of blood, Swallowing (difficult), Throat (inflammation of the), Tonsillitis, Tracheal irritation, Tracheitis, Vocal cord (inflammation of the), Voice (loss of).

Pettorale 2.

Angina in the chest, Aphonia, Bronchitis (capillary), Cavities in the lungs, with *Canc.*, Congestion of the lungs, Cough with fœtid breath, Cough with greenish expectoration, Croup, Emphysema (pulmonary), Hæmorrhage of the lungs, with *Ang.*, Inflammation of the lungs, Laryngeal pain in speaking, Laryngitis (chronic, even with ulceration), Phthisis, with loss of voice and vomiting of food, Phthisis (tubercular, slow or galloping, with *Canc.*), Pneumonia (with hæmorrhage), Pneumonia (chronic), Pneumorrhagia (symptomatic of tubercular fusion), Pulmonary cavities, with *Canc.*, Pulmonary inflammation, Pulmonary flux, symptomatic of tubercular softening.

Pettorale 3.

The gentlest of all, therefore best suited to children. Catarrh (chronic), Catarrh (suffocating, of the aged), Bronchial catarrh (acute and chronic), Cough (all kinds), Cough, with yellowish expectoration and cold in the head, Children's chest complaints, Pains in the chest (cramping and constrictive).

Pettorale 4.

Asthma, Bronchial dilatation, Bronchial catarrh (chronic), Croup, Laryngeal phthisis, Mucus in the larynx, causing constant expectoration, Phthisis in the second stage, Pulmonary catarrh (chronic), Sharp pains in the chest.

Linfatico.

This remedy occupies a position between the *Angioiticos* and the *Scrofolosos*, and is chiefly used in ointments, frictions, compresses and baths. Internally it is used for Angina Pectoris, Asthma (catarrhal), Cephalalgia (tractive), Colic at the periods, Congestion and hardening of the glands, Creeping sensation in the skin with pruritus and desquammation. Fistula (dental), Gastric debility, Gastric fevers, with *Feb.*, Generative debility, Glandular enlargement with induration, Gout, Fits of insanity and mania, Hæmorrhoids (blind and fluent), Headache, Intermittent fever, with *Feb.*, Kidney diseases, Lymphatic complaints of children, Memory (weakness of), Menstruation, with colic before or after), Muscular weakness, Perspiration of the feet (excessive), Prostrate fluid (flow of at stool), Rheumatic fevers, with *Feb.*, Testicles (inflammation of), Toothache, Vertigo (with nausea), Weakness in pit of stomach (sensation of).

Venereo.

A remedy which has remarkable effects in all primary, secondary, tertiary and even hereditary venereal cases, Angina (syphilitic), Blenorrhagia, Blenorrhœa, Bone (caries of, syphilitic), Bubo (congested glands in the groin, anus, &c.), Chordee, Cockscombs, Condyloma, Chancres (simple, indurated, soft), Congenital syphilis, Conjunctiva (syphilitic), Eczema (syphilitic), Exostosis (syphilitic), Gonorrhœa, Iritis (syphilitic), Leucorrhœa (obstinate), Mercurial diseases, Neuralgia (syphilitic), Nocturnal osseous pains, Nose (caries of the bone) Ophthalmia (syphilitic), Orchitis (syphilitic), Palate (caries of the bone of), Phymosis, Primary syphilis, during period of incubation *Scrof. 1* is necessary, Rheumatism (gonorrhœal), Stricture (gonorrhœal), Syphilitic ulcerations, with *Canc.*, Sycosis, Throat (ulceration, when syphilitic), Ulcerations (venereal), Urethral inflammation (syphilitic), Vaginal inflammation (syphilitic), Venereal consumption.

Vermifugo 1.

Specific against worms of all kinds; also useful in many nervous affections.

Ascarides, Cramp in stomach, Diarrhœa (through worms), Epilepsy, Hyponchondriasis, Hysteria, Indigestion, Insomnia (through worms), Intestinal worms, Lumbricoides, Melancholia, Nausea (through worms), Thread worms, Tænia, Tricocephalus, Worm fever.

Vermifugo 2.

Used as an injection (20 globules with 10 drops of *Yellow* electricity) or in ointments and compresses as an adjuvant to *Ver 1*.

Anti-Mal de Mer.

Useful for preventing and curing Sea-sickness.

Domfin.

Specific for Diphtheria. Valuable in almost all kinds of Throat Disease.

Marina.

Valuable in the treatment of most forms of acute and chronic Eye Diseases.

II.—THE ELECTRICITIES.

These mysterious liquids, which baffle analysis, act with remarkable power and promptitude. Count Mattei strongly believes that he has discovered a method of charging liquids with various forms of vegetable electricity. The possibility of doing this is more easily believed in now that scientists, like Prof. Crookes, are asserting that there are electrical as there are chemical atoms. These electric liquids are chiefly used externally. In some cases, however, they are taken internally, in doses varying from $\frac{1}{10}$ of a drop, in the case of *Green* Electricity, to 4 and 5 drops in the case of *Red*, *White*, *Blue* and *Yellow* Electricities.

The liquids were originally coloured. Now, however, they are colourless. They are distinguished by the variously coloured labels on the bottles in which they are sold.

1.—Red Electricity (Positive).

This has a positive action. It stimulates vitality and increases the rapidity of the circulation. On this account it is suited to persons of lymphatic temperament. In cases of severe erysipelas it may be successfully applied to the forehead and to the places marked 1, 2, 12, 18 in the diagram. It is also useful when applied to the affected portions of the body on its negative parts, or on its central lines in cases of Chills, Colds in the head, Deafness (nervousness), Debility (general), Difficult child-birth,

Hemiplegia, Pains arising from bruises, contusions, &c., Pains in the womb, Sciatica (apply to hollow of foot), Semi-anchylosis, Sight (weakness of), Tic-douloureux.

Two to five drops of *Red* Electricity on sugar, or in a dessert spoonful of water, sometimes serve as a good tonic for lymphatic patients. Gargles of *Red* Electricity are useful in some throat cases.

Red Electricity should not be applied to wounds.

2.—Yellow Electricity (Negative).

This has a negative action, and checks excess of vitality. After applying *Red* Electricity, equilibrium may be restored by the use of *Yellow* Electricity. This Electricity relaxes Muscular tension, and has removed partial Tetanus, Trismus, Cramp, &c. Taken internally in one or two drops it will often relieve stomachic pains. It lessens Muscular contraction, Nervous irritability, and has even been recommended for the treatment of Fevers.

In larger doses (5 drops) it serves as a drastic purgative and vermifuge.

Count Mattei advises the application of *Yellow* (negative) Electricity to the positive and central parts of the body, when these are painful, in cases of Deafness (nervous), Hemiplegia, Pains arising from bruises, Pains in the womb (apply to the left sacral nerve), Sciatica (apply to the points where the sciatic nerve issues), Semi-anchylosis, Tic-douloureux.

When applied to the central parts of the body the *Yellow* Electricity should be used two or three seconds after the *Red*.

Yellow Electricity should not be applied to wounds.

3.—Blue Electricity. (Positive.)

This liquid is used in the same diseases as *Red* Electricity, for patients of sanguine temperaments, for whom *Red* is too stimulating. It has bracing properties. It stimulates those nerves which control the circulatory system, and is, therefore, useful in the treatment of all diseases of the blood and blood vessels, especially in hæmorrhage and varices.

The external application of Blue Electricity to a dog on one occasion caused greatly quickened breathing.

It is useful in regulating menstruation, checking chills and allaying pulmonary congestion. It stops palpitation and gives tone to the heart when applied over that organ by means of small compresses moistened with from 5 to 10 drops of it. Burning cancer pains may be relieved by this Electricity, applied in the same way, in somewhat larger doses (10 to 20 drops).

4.—White Electricity. (Neutral.)

This is neutral and suited to all temperaments. It is specially serviceable in removing pains in the abdomen, head and womb. Like *Blue* Electricity it may be used to assist hæmorrhage. It may advantageously be applied to sores and relieves intermittent neuralgic pains in cancers, &c. Internally it is useful in Arthritis, Balanitis, Gastritis, Inflammation of the intestines, Mesenteritis, Meningitis, Megrim, Muscular diseases, Neuralgia, Œsophagitis, Orchitis, Ovaritis, Peritonitis, Pharyngitis, Pneumonia, Stomatitis, Tuberculosis, Visceral diseases.

5.—Green Electricity. (Negative.)

This has attained special renown because of its remarkable power of dispelling lancinating pain in Cancers, Sores, Ulcers, &c. It is also useful in allaying articular (joint) pains. It has the power of promoting cicatrization.

POINTS TO WHICH ELECTRICITIES SHOULD BE APPLIED.

(See Diagram at the end of the book.)

On points along the central line of the body use the Positive and Negative Electricities in succession, after a few seconds' interval. On other points apply Positive Electricity to negative parts, and *vice-versâ*. *White* Electricity may be applied to any point.

When the Electricities are applied pure it is often advisable to moisten the tip of the finger with the fluid and to gently rub the points indicated for about 10 seconds each.

To act on the Arm.—Brachial Nerve.

Bladder.—Perineum, Pubes, Sacral Nerves (both right and left sides), Coccyx.

Body (whole).—Occiput, Solar Plexus, Pit of Stomach, Great Sympathetic (both sides).

Ears.—Cavity of Ear, under Ear in hollow near Jaw.

Eyes.—Occiput, Temples. Back of neck. Super and sub-orbitals.

Face.—Under the ear, Suborbitals.

Forehead—Superorbitals, Temples.

Head.—Nape of Neck, Root of Nose, Temples, Crown of Head.

Heart.— Solar Plexus, Sympathetic. Pass a few drops lightly over the Heart.

Intestines.—Solar Plexus. Gastric sympathetic. Also (mixed with a little glycerine and spirit) over lower abdomen.

Leg.—Points of Sciatic and Crural Nerves. In cavity above and below the knee. Soles of Feet.

Liver. — Solar Plexus. Also over hypochondriac region, in liniment with *Feb. 2.*

Lungs.—Solar Plexus, Also over chest, in liniment with *Pet.* or *Canc.*

Nose.—Root of Nose, Nasal nerves (each side).

Sexual Organs.—Pubes, Perineum, Sacral Nerves.

Spleen.—Solar Plexus. Also liniment with *Feb.* over region of spleen.

Stomach.— Pit of Stomach, Bottom of Stomach, Gastric Sympathetic Nerve.

Tongue.—Large and small Hypoglossi (both sides).

Womb. — Pubes, Perineum, Sacral Nerves (both sides).

INTERNAL USE OF THE ELECTRICITIES

These are chiefly used externally. In some cases, however, they may be taken internally either on sugar or in a dessertspoonful of water. The addition of a little spirit or glycerine is believed, by at least one careful Mattei practitioner, to enhance the effect. The doses may be repeated from once a day to once an hour, according to the nature of the case.

(1) **Red Electricity** is highly stimulating and greatly quickens the circulation. It is, therefore, unwise for patients of a sanguine temperament to make use of it. The proper dose is from 1 to 5 drops.

It should be proved that *Red* Electricity agrees externally before it is given internally. Indeed this principle applies to each of the Electricities.

(2) **Blue Electricity** also has a tonic effect, but it does not excite the circulatory system like *Red* Electricity. On the contrary it calms it when it has been over stimulated. It contracts relaxed blood vessels, and is therefore valuable in the treatment of varices. It has been found useful in cases of sanguine apoplexy, in which as many as fifty drops have been used with beneficial results. In cases of arterial hæmorrhage it may be given in two drop doses every half hour. In cerebral congestion, buzzing in the ears, &c., it may be taken in 2 to 5 drop doses every hour. Hysterical patients, of sanguine temperament,

may take 2 drops of *Blue* Electricity twice a day. Some patients, however, cannot take a single drop without discomfort.

(3) **Yellow Electricity** relaxes muscular or nervous tension, lowers excessive vitality, and diminishes nervous excitement. It may, therefore, be used by patients of lymphatic temperament who suffer from hysteria and tetanus. In cases of extreme nervous tension it affords relief if taken in 1 to 3 drop doses. It is valuable as a vermifuge, and may be used for this purpose in 1 to 5 drop doses. As a drastic purgative, which should only be resorted to in exceptional circumstances, it may be administered in 3 to 8 drop doses. It must not, on any account, be used when there is any tendency to hæmorrhage.

(4) **White Electricity** exerts a gentle calming influence over the nervous system, which is of special value in cases of congestion, inflammation or fever. The doses vary from 1 to 5 drops. In one singular instance the enormous dose of 100 drops, taken by mistake, by a victim of arthritis, produced remarkable relief.

(5) **Green Electricity** has lately been tried internally for the relief of the pains of internal cancer. It must, however, be very cautiously administered. A single drop should be added to a quart of water, and this "electrified" water should be taken in spoonfuls at hourly or half-hourly intervals. Should colicky pains follow its use it may be concluded that the dose is too strong, or that it is being too frequently repeated.

When taking *Blue*, *Red*, *White* or *Yellow* Electricities internally it is well to begin with a one drop dose, and to increase the dose gradually as the patient is able to bear it.

The use of a tube dropper is recommended, as accurate measurement is highly important.

EXTERNAL USE OF THE GLOBULES.

Any of the globules may be used externally in baths, compresses, &c. Those, however, which are most frequently so used are the following:

(1) **Canceroso 5,** which is beneficial in all deep-seated disorders of the absorbent and vascular systems, and is singularly useful in the treatment of Syphilitic ailments. It is also highly serviceable in Eczema and other cutaneous disorders.

(2) **Scrofoloso 5** — valuable in Gout, glandular diseases, and chronic skin diseases (for some of which, however, it is better to begin with *Scrofoloso 1*).

(3) **Angioitico 3**—serviceable in all disorders of the circulatory system. Compresses of *Ang. 3*, applied to painful parts, will often afford relief when the Electricities have failed to do so, owing to the pain having originated in vascular disturbance. At other times they will prepare

time it is necessary to add fresh supplies of hot water from time to time in order that the temperature of the bath may be kept up. Care should be taken not to take a chill after coming out of a warm bath. The patient should be dried with a long sheet or bath towel, and well wrapped in a warm blanket immediately afterwards. Baths of *Linfatico* and *Angioitico* do not generally require to be as strong as others. *Canc. 5* baths are found by some persons to be very exciting.

Sitz Bath. This is best taken in a bath specially made for the purpose. The patient sits in it, sometimes with his feet in another small bath filled with hot water. The water should be about 4 inches deep. A bath with a double bottom, the upper one being perforated, is useful, inasmuch as it admits of fresh supplies of water being poured in without disturbing the patient. Hot sitz baths help in restoring menstruation. Cool sitz baths are useful in dysmenorrhœa. Piles, weakness of the sexual organs, &c., may be treated by means of these baths, many of which may be medicated with from 25 to 50 globules.

2. **Compress.** There are three classes of compresses (*a*) the heating or stimulating compress, (*b*) the cooling compress and (*c*) the medicating compress. The *stimulating compress* is prepared by wringing out a piece of lint or linen which has been dipped in water, placing outside this a piece of gutta percha or oiled silk, which should be a quarter of an inch larger every way than the lint, and binding the whole together with flannel. Spongio-piline sometimes answers well for a compress, when the skin is not inflamed nor tender. Its size and shape varies according as it is to be worn over the throat, the chest,

the heart, or the abdomen. The cooling compress, which is extremely valuable in fevers and during dentition, is made by taking a strip of linen broad enough to reach from below the armpit to the waist, and long enough to encircle the body, wringing this out of water and wrapping round it two folds of dry linen. Care must be taken that compresses are thoroughly wrung out. The cooling compress becomes doubly valuable if the water used is previously medicated with Febrifugo 2 globules and White Electricity. The *medicating compress* may be made either with or without waterproof material. If it has oiled silk over it, and is bound on closely, or kept in place by the clothing it will keep warm and moist for several hours. It should be taken off before it becomes dry. The lint which has been removed should be well rinsed out of boiling water. If a compress is made of old linen, this should be soaked in boiling water so as to remove any soap or soda which may remain in it.

A thick covering of flannel alone should be used if oiled silk causes irritation, and always over open wounds. The medicated lotions for moistening the compresses, when waterproof material is used aud the compress is thus a heating compress, are usually made by dissolving 10 to 20 globules in a tumbler of water. These should be changed as soon as dry. If no waterproof material is used a larger number of globules (30 to 40) may be used. Lotions for Compresses may be kept ready-made in a bottle. 3 or 4 globules may be allowed for each ounce of water. If Electricity is added the proportion is 1 drop to each globule. As a rule it is better to use the warm compress for the throat and the cool compress for the head, eyes, and legs.

3. **Body Pack.** This is very useful in gastric and other fevers. Take a sheet. Dip it in a bucket of water in which a few (20 to 25) globules of Febrifugo 2 have been dissolved. Wring it thoroughly out by means of a mangle or wringer. Lay it on a bed, over which a waterproof sheet and a couple of blankets have been spread. Smooth it well out. Then lay the patient naked on this sheet, which should project beyond his feet. Take hold of one side of the sheet, and, raising his arms, wrap this side tightly over the body and tuck it under the opposite side of the body. Then place his arms along his sides, tuck the other side of the sheet over the arms and body, and turn the projecting ends over the feet. (In some cases, however, it is better to leave the feet projecting beyond the sheet, and to apply hot bottles to them). Then tuck the upper part of the sheet tightly over the patient's shoulders, tuck the blankets well over his feet, sides and neck, so as to entirely exclude the cold air, and put a stout quilt or extra blanket over all. After a while the patient will feel very comfortable and may even fall asleep. It is usual to give him draughts of cold water while he is in the pack. Sips of Febrifugo 1 in the second or third dilution would be very useful. After he has been in the pack from 30 to 60 minutes he should stand on a hot pad laid in a shallow bath, be well sponged over with vinegar and tepid water, dried rapidly with a very large bath sheet or towel and put to bed. A compress wrung out of a quarter of a pint of cold water in which two globules of Angioitico 3 have been dissolved, may be applied to the forehead during

the packing to relieve congestion.

4. **Half-pack, Towel-pack or Fever Compress.** This is a very valuable modification of the preceding, and is extremely useful in the treatment of fevers. The plan adopted is to take a strip of calico, linen, or a towel, wring it thoroughly out of water, medicated with Febrifugo 2, as before. Wrap this tightly round the trunk of the body and put a protecting bandage outside it.

5. **Fomentations.** These are invaluable in the treatment of disorders of the liver and stomach, and especially when medicated with the appropriate globules or electricities. A thick piece of flannel is tightly folded into two or three times its original thickness. This pad is then dipped into a bucketful of boiling water which has been duly medicated and wrung out. As the latter part of the process exposes the attendant to the risk of scalding himself it is well to wring out the foment-flannel in a thick towel by holding the ends of the latter and twisting them in opposite directions. The foment pad is then applied to the part which it is desired to treat. It is a good plan to keep up the heat by means of a fomenting can filled with boiling water, or by means of spongio-piline, which may be laid over the pad. If there be no such appliance at hand the compress should be well wrapped round with flannel and kept on for a few minutes, but not after it becomes sensibly cool.

6. **Vapour Bath.** This is very serviceable in the treatment of some forms of rheumatism and skin disease. It is best taken in a specially prepared apparatus. But it may also be taken in the following way: Take a cane-seat chair. Place a piece of flannel over it. Seat the patient

upon this. Tie a crinoline-like frame over him and the chair. Over this fasten blankets in such a way that when they are let down they will keep in the steam about to be introduced beneath the chair. Then set a bucket of boiling water beneath the chair, taking care that the surface of the water is not so near the seat that the steam will scald the patient. Then let the blankets down and allow him to be bathed in steam for 10 to 15 minutes. Should it be needful, it is easy to produce a fresh supply of steam, by gently plunging a hot brick or heated iron into the water. It is a good plan to place the patient's feet in hot water and to give him sips of cold water during the bath. A head band, wrung out of cold water, may be worn around the forehead. After the steaming the patient should be rapidly bathed with tepid water, well dried, and put to bed.

7. **The Hot Air Bath** is similar to this. In this case, however, instead of producing steam, we simply produce hot air. This is done by placing a spirit lamp, or a saucer containing one or two ounces of spirits of wine, on the floor beneath the chair, and igniting it. The patient, wrapped in blankets as before, is soon surrounded by so hot a layer of air that he perspires profusely. On coming out he should be sponged and well dried, as in the preceding cases.

8. **Eyewash.**—Dissolve 2 to 3 globules in a Collyrium eye-glassful of tepid water, and bathe the eye with this once or twice a day. Or take a one ounce phial. Half fill this with boiled water. Drop into the water 10 globules of *Marina*. When they are thoroughly dissolved add 10 drops of pure spirit. Soak a piece of lint in hot water and wring it well out or warm the lint before

the fire. Then moisten it thoroughly with the eye lotion and lay it over the closed lids. Should this cause smarting add a little water to the lotion.

9. **Gargles.**—The proportions of the remedies used for medicating water for gargling are from 10 to 20 globules, or 8 to 10 drops of Electricity, to a tumblerful of water. Use from two to three times a day, or oftener if it is found beneficial to do so.

10. **Injections.**—Dissolve 5 to 15 globules in, or add 1 teaspoonful of Electricity to, three-quarters of a tumblerful of tepid water. Use once a day.

11. **Inhalations and Sprays.**—Same proportions.

12. **Lotions.**—Dissolve from 10 to 30 globules in, or add 1 desertspoonful of Electricity to, an eight ounce bottleful of water. To keep the lotion from spoiling, it is advisable to add a tablespoonful of proof spirit or eau-de-cologne, but it is better to use pure water than to add any adulterated spirit. When baths cannot be taken, the whole body may be well rubbed over with a towel soaked in a suitable lotion.

13. **Oils.**—Made by dissolving 10 to 20 globules in a few drops of hot water in a bottle and adding one ounce of sweet oil. Shake thoroughly before using. Rub two or three times a day.

14. **Ointments.**— Made by dissolving 10 to 20 globules in half a drachm or a quarter of a teaspoonful of water or the appropriate Electricity, and, when quite dissolved, beating thoroughly well up with one ounce of lanoline, white vaseline, fresh lard or other pure ointment. (*Scrof.* dissolved in *Red* Electricity, *Feb.* or *Linf.* in *White*, *Canc.* dissolved in *Green* Electricity, *Ang.* in *Blue*). Apply once

or twice a day. These Ointments can be obtained ready made at the various Mattei depôts.

15. **Suppositories** made of *Canc. 5* and *Green* El. are also obtainable, and are useful in cancer of the rectum or of the uterus. Similar suppositories of *Ang. 2* or *3* and *Blue* El. are valuable accessories in the treatment of hæmorrhage, piles and obstinate constipation. Before introducing the suppositories they should be well lubricated with pure olive oil.

V.—HOW TO SELECT THE REMEDIES.

IN order that the right remedy may be applied it is necessary that the real disease should be discovered. True diagnosis must precede successful treatment. And no diagnosis can be considered to be both true and complete which simply or even chiefly takes cognizance of a local ailment. The state of the whole organism must be ascertained and noted. For it must always be remembered that it is more important to cure a constitutional disease than to dispel one or more of its local symptoms, that if the roots be extirpated the branches will soon wither, but that if the branch alone is cut down, while the root is left, it is extremely probable that it will soon put forth new shoots. On this account it has been necessary to lay down the law that the selection of the remedies to be given to a particular patient must be determined, not so much by the nature of the local disease from which he is suffering, as by the general constitutional state in which he is found.

1. A person of a *sanguine* or *angioitic temperament* will need to be treated with one of the *Angioitics*, especially *Ang. 3*. The characteristic marks of the temperament which needs these remedies are chiefly the following:—

Rapid circulation, great sensitiveness, lively disposition, florid complexion, smooth skin, tendency to palpitation, tendency to bleeding piles, tendency to congestion, tendency to hæmorrhage, tendency to varicose veins, tendency to vertigo, tendency to sleeplessness. tendency to inflammatory throat and chest diseases, obstinate constipation.

In females : Early and profuse menstruation.

Persons of this temperament should avoid *Red* Electricity and *Scrof. 1*. They may use *Scrof. 2.*

2. A person of *lymphatic temperament* will require *Scrof. 1*. The lymphatic temperament is characterised by the following features :—

Sluggish circulation, pale face, except when hectic appears, slow digestion, poor appetite, frequent colds, heavy sleep, tendency to glandular swellings, tendency to skin eruptions.

In females : Suppressed menses, or tendency to suppressed menstruation, Leucorrhœa, Chlorosis.

3. A person of *nervous temperament* will require both *Ang. 3* and *Scrof. 1*. The characteristic marks of this temperament are :—

Thready and frequent pulse, thinness, soft muscles, pale colour, great excitability, strong emotions, studious disposition, tendency to nervous palpitation.

Persons of this temperament will be extremely susceptible to the action of the remedies, and should use small doses. *Feb. 1* will be of great service to them, and baths of *Feb. 2* will calm them when unduly excited.

4. A person of *bilious* temperament will require *Angioitico 1* and *Scrofoloso 5*, combined with frequent

doses of *Feb. 1* and the external use of *Feb. 2*. *Scrof. 1* does not suit bilious people. The marks of the bilious temperament are the following:—Dark hair, yellowish skin, firmly developed muscles, irritability, tenacity.

Patients of mixed temperaments must combine the treatments adapted to the types which are mingled together in their constitution in the proportion in which they are so mingled.

If in the case of a patient of any one of these temperaments the disease has reached so grave a stage that it fails to yield to the ordinary constitutional treatment, it is necessary to call in the aid of one of the *Anticancerosos* or of *Anti-Venereo* if the presence of some syphilitic taint is suspected.

As in many cases the curative process is hindered by the presence of Ascarides or other internal parasites, the great worm specifics *Vermifugo 1* and *2* and *Yellow* Electridity should be tried in all instances where the ordinary treatment fails.

In all cases where the chest is attacked it is necessary to combine the use of one or more of the *Pettorales* with the remedies suited to the patient's constitutional condition, and wherever there is any unnatural elevation of the bodily temperature, the *Febrifugos* must be used both internally and externally. If the throat is affected, *Dom Fin* will be found exceedingly useful. And in most eye diseases *Marina* will be of considerable service.

Patients who have been subjected to previous drug treatment will find it advantageous to take 3 globules of *Scrofoloso 5* several times daily, in chronic cases, until some effect is observed.

It is important to remember that *Scrofoloso* subdues inflammations; that *Angioitico* relieves congestions, and that *Linfatico* serves as a tonic to the vaso-motor system.

It may be noted that *Angioitico 3* or *2* ointment, used externally, often paves the way for applying the Electricities or suitable compresses.

In the dictionary of diseases, at the end of this book, there is given a list of the remedies which have been found most useful in the treatment of particular complaints. Those who use this list should not allow themselves to become slaves to it. What is one man's meat is another man's poison. The remedy which has cured nine persons of a certain disease may altogether fail to relieve a tenth person, who is suffering from the same complaint. Aided, however, by the principles just laid down, it will soon become easy to select the most suitable remedy for most cases. In some instances, however, it will be difficult, and considerable patience will have to be exercised. In these cases it will be well to try successively the other remedies in the particular group which seems most suited to the patient's constitution. After trying *Ang. 3* try *Ang. 2* and then *Ang. 1*. After trying *Canc. 1* try *Canc. 2*, *Canc. 4*, *Canc. 5*, or if you fear that *Canc. 1* has been too strong a remedy try *Canc. 6*. After trying *Scrof. 1* try *Scrof. 5* or *Scrof. 2*. Sometimes recourse may be had to *Linfatico*, which occasionally produces surprisingly good effects.

HOW TO COMBINE THE REMEDIES.

It has already been observed that some of the remedies, such as *Scrofoloso*, *Canceroso*, and *Angioitico* have a general constitutional action, and that others, such as *Pettorale*, have a special action on certain organs. The question will frequently present itself whether the special remedy, the constitutional remedy, or a combination of both should be used. The following hints may guide inquirers to the solution of the problem :—

1st—When, as in an attack of diphtheria, the local affection demands prompt treatment, and threatens to take away life if that treatment is not given, the special remedy must be diligently applied until the alarming symptoms have passed away. Even in this case, however, care must be taken to regulate the functions generally.

2nd—When there is no special disorder, but simply a condition of general ill-health, the constitutional remedy best adapted to the patient's temperament should be used.

3rd—In all other cases the constitutional and special remedy should be combined, in the proportions which best harmonise with the patient's state.

In most instances the first remedy indicated soon produces a condition in which some other remedy also becomes necessary.

In selecting the constitutional remedy, it is highly important to remember that *Ang. 3*, is the remedy for persons of sanguine temperament, but that it should be alternated with *Canc. 1*, whenever the patient's state is decidedly grave; that *Scrof. 5*, is the remedy for bilious temperaments as well as for all persons who suffer from skin eruptions of a chronic character, and that *Canceroso* should be combined with or take the place of the *Scrofolosos* whenever the disease is so profoundly seated that it will resist the action of the *Scrofolosos*. This happens in all cases of suppuration and glandular induration.

VI.—HOW TO DETERMINE THE DOSE.

1. Dilutions.

ALMOST, if not quite, equal in importance to the selection of the right remedy is the discovery of the right dose. And it is by no means child's play to ascertain this. Both careful observation and patient waiting may be necessary ere this extremely important problem has been solved. The doses suggested in the handbooks will not suit all classes of patients. Age, sex, temperament, climate, and a host of other things, affect the sensitiveness of sufferers. It would seem, for instance, that English people are peculiarly susceptible to the influence of the *Angioiticos* and of *Linfatico*. And it is of the first importance to proportion the dose to the patient's sensitiveness. The more highly sensitive a patient is, either naturally or in consequence of his present or past experiences, or environment, the weaker will be the dose which is necessary to produce a given effect upon him. Thus it happens that persons who are naturally extremely nervous, or who are suffering from high fever, hysteria, or organic heart disease, generally find that the third dilution is quite strong enough for them. Infants and little children, too, need no stronger remedy. But in the case of those who are less sensitive, the second, intermediate, or even first dilutions, may produce the best effects.

What is known as the litre or intermediate dilution is most generally useful. This, as will be shown subsequently, is made by dissolving 1 globule, *i.e.*, one little pill, in a litre (1⅞ pints) of water. In the vast majority of diseases adults may first make use of the litre dilution. Should this produce any discomfort, they should substitute for it the second dilution, and should this still cause any unpleasant sensation, or aggravate any of the symptoms of disease, they must make use of the third dilution if they wish to obtain a cure as speedily as possible. If on the other hand the litre dilution produces no effects whatever, the first dilution should be used.

Various intermediate dilutions may be tried in addition to that to which we have given this name, *e.g.*, 1 globule to a pint, 1 globule to 2 quarts, &c.

Ladies should not discontinue the remedies during the monthly illness.

In selecting the dose it is essential to remember that it has been found that sometimes different dilutions produce altogether different and even opposite effects. This discovery harmonises with the fact that the effects of a strong current of electricity on the motor nerves are usually opposite to the effects of a weak current. It has been noticed, for instance, that the *Angioiticos* in the first dilution increase the rapidity of the circulation, and so restore periodical functions which have been arrested, but that in the third dilution they diminish the speed of the circulation and check or arrest congestions or any excessive periodical functions. *Scrofoloso* in the first dilution will throw out a skin eruption which has been suppressed, and is therefore useful in the first stage of eruptive fevers. On this account, however, it must be avoided in eczema, and the second or third dilution which gently disperses the eruption, must be used instead.

Patients who suffer from Aneurism, Convulsions, Hysteria, or Organic Heart Disease, should take either the third dilution or at most three or four teaspoonfuls of the litre or second dilution per diem.

Indeed it is often better to begin the treatment of these diseases with ointments only, next to use dry globules, and only afterwards to proceed to use the third dilution.

In the case of infants and children the following rules may be followed:

1. Sucklings can best be treated through their mothers, who should take the same dose as if they themselves were suffering from their infants' malady. Infants brought up by hand require the third dilution. Sometimes, however, it is best to put the globules into their food in the proportion of 5 globules to a quart.

2. From 2 to 6. Take ¼ of a tumblerful of the dilution which would be given to a similar adult in a similar condition; add this to ¾ of a tumblerful of water and give teaspoonfuls of this during the day. Or give the ¼ tumblerful pure in 15 drop doses.

3. From 6 to 12. Take ½ tumblerful as above or give 30 drop (½ teaspoonful) doses.

An alternative method is suggested in the Table of Doses.

2. Dry Globules.

When it is impossible to take the dilutions a dry globule of the remedy prescribed in dilution may be taken every hour or even every half-hour, during that part of the day for which it is prescribed. Or three to five globules may be taken dry on the tongue night and morning, immediately after each meal, or in the beverage at meals. Massive doses act more promptly than minute doses, and are, therefore, preferable in cases where immediate results are required. In Fainting fits, Cramp, Paralysis, Seasickness, accumulation of mucous in the bronchial tubes, arrested suppuration, Chills, &c., massive doses are useful. But as all abnormal action is followed by a corresponding reaction, it is far better to use minute doses in the treatment of chronic diseases. A massive dose (5 to 10 globules) of *Pettorale* will promote expectoration and so relieve the bronchial tubes; 5 globules of *Vermifugo* will put an end to Nervous Attacks, Partial Contractions, Cramps of the Stomach and Womb; 5 globules of *Scrofoloso* will restore the faint, relieve Cramp, &c.; 2 to 5 globules of *Angioitico* will quicken the circulation, bring on suppressed menses, and take the place of brandy in cases of failure of the heart's action. The action of the last named remedy renders it unsafe for persons subject to hæmorrhage to take more than one dry globule at a time.

The Doses used for external treatment should be proportionate to those used internally, as shown in the following:

TABLE OF DOSES.

SUITED TO DIFFERENT PERSONS.

	Infants.	*Children under 8 years Epileptical & Hysterical Patients. Patients in High Fever.*	*Children from 2 to 6. Patients in Fever.*	*Children from 6 to 12 and very Sensitive Women.*	*Women and very Sensitive Men.*	*Men.*
Dilutions	III. in ½ tea-spoonfuls.	III. 8 teasp'nfuls per diem.	III.	II.	I.	I. or pint dilution.
Globules in beverage at Meals	One small sized glob.	1 Globule	2	3	4	5
Dry Globules night & morning	ditto	1 Globule	2	3	4—5	5—10
Dry Globules.. ..	Once a day	Twice a day	4 times a day	6 times a day	8 times a day	Hourly
Globules to 6 ounces of water for making lotions for compresses, inhalations, injections.	5	7	10	15	18	20
Globules to ounce for Ointments	5	7	10	15	18	20
Globules for Bath ..	5 (small bath)	7 (small bath)	40 (full body bath	60	75	100
Globules for Sitz Baths			15	20	25	30

As the disease yields to the action of the remedies the doses must be gradually increased, but the increase must never be carried to such a degree as to produce discomfort or aggravating symptoms.

In some cases, however, especially after drug treatment, or when the functions are sluggish, the doses have to be massive at first, and must be gradually attenuated as sensitiveness becomes apparent.

In selecting the dose the climate must be considered. *In warm weather, or when there is much electricity in the air, smaller doses must be given than in cold weather.*

It is well to know precisely what are the symptoms of an over-dose. For very frequently after a right remedy has been found the selection of too strong a dose causes waste of time and disappointment to the patient, even if it does not lead him to lose faith in the remedies. *Angioitico* quickens the circulation, and therefore, an overdose of it will lead to symptoms of congestion in the head, throbbing in the temples, buzzing in the ears, palpitation and sometimes even vertigo and bleeding from the nose. An overdose of *Scrofoloso* may produce wakefulness, constipation in sanguine patients, and diarrhœa in lymphatic patients. An overdose of *Vermifugo* will produce pain in the abdomen, nervous agitation and diarrhœa. An overdose of *Canceroso* will have a similar effect to that produced by *Scrofoloso.* An overdose of *Venereo* will bring out an eruption on the skin. And, generally, it may be stated that an overdose of any remedy will aggravate the symptoms which that remedy rightly taken is best calculated to relieve.

When an overdose has been taken its effects may, in

some cases, be counteracted by a few dry globules of *Scrofoloso*, in others by the third dilution of the remedy which has produced unpleasant effects, and in all by a teaspoonful of lemon juice. The latter, however, may render the subsequent treatment ineffective for a time.

MINUTE DOSES.

In experimenting with his remedies Count Mattei discovered that minute doses were generally the best and that it was usually necessary that the dose should be in inverse ratio to the gravity of the disease. In treating a high fever he found it needful to use a high dilution. This led him to conclude that atomic forces come into play when matter is detached from its massive aggregations in which these forces exist in a latent state.

Other explanations have been given of the fact that the diseases by which the organism is evidently greatly disturbed require minute doses. The writer, for instance, believes that the symptoms of disease are often the outward and visible signs of the effort which nature is making to rid herself of some foe, and that as a rule the stronger the effort that nature is making the more serious the symptoms appear. It is when the air currents are running most rapidly that wrecks strew our coast. Now as the Mattei medicines act homœopathically, in the same direction as nature, and not, allopathically, in the contrary direction, it seems reasonable to suppose that the addition of a small amount of energy to that which is already at work will suffice to produce the desired effect. When a train is on the track it may need an enormous force to set it going at the rate of one mile per hour. But when once it has started it needs comparatively little force to add a mile per hour to its speed. And the quicker it is travelling the less is the force required. If, however, it is desired to act allopathically against the impetus which the train has acquired, it needs comparatively little force to stop it at the start, but the faster it is going the greater is the force needed. Those who have been accustomed to work against the forces of nature do not realise how different a thing it is to work with them. To row a mile with the tide is a very different thing from rowing a mile against it. If Cleopatra's needle were detached from its base, and were standing in a state of unstable equilibrium, a child's push might cast it to the ground. But it would need enormous leverage to lift it up again. Such is the difference between homœopathy and allopathy. The former works with the forces which the body brings into play. The latter struggles against them. The former drives disease back. The latter helps nature to drive it out.

Those who deny the possibility of producing curative effects by means of such minute doses as are often employed by homœopaths and electro-homœopaths prove by so doing that they have never seriously studied the power of the infinitely little. If any of them should read these pages they are invited to carefully consider the following truths :—

1. That many scientists are strongly inclined to believe with Professor Graham, that not only are all bodies built up of atoms, but that the ultimate atoms of all bodies are alike.

2. That, although it is generally believed that the

ultimate atoms are grouped together in various ways to form molecules of various elements, and that these molecules are incapable of being broken up by any known forces, there are many who hope to discover a way of reducing the molecules back to their ultimate atoms, of again re-building the molecules from those ultimate atoms, and thus of turning any element into any other element, thereby realising the ideal of the alchemist who hoped to turn the baser metals into gold.

3. That it has been proved that the diameter of the ultimate atoms cannot be more than $\frac{1}{250000000}$ of an inch.

4. That, therefore, the atoms are so small that at least 15,625,000,000,000,000,000,000 could be packed into a cubic inch of space, and that it is probable that a very much larger number could be compressed into this area.

5. That one of Count Mattei's globules of Scrofoloso in comparison with an atom of matter is as a massive mountain compared with a small fragment of rock.

6. That chemical changes take place through the action of molecules upon molecules or atoms upon atoms, and not simply through the action of a mass of molecules upon another mass.

7. That one form of matter is free to unite itself with other forms in proportion as it becomes attenuated, or, in other words, in proportion as its molecular masses become detached from each other. The chemist who wishes to make two substances re-act upon each other finds that they do so with incomparably more force when they are dissolved in a liquid than when they are left in the solid state. Heat increases the possibility of forming new chemical compounds by placing a greater distance between the mole-

cules and so giving them freer play. The truth thus illustrated may partly account for a fact which puzzles so many Matteists, viz., that A TEASPOONFUL OF THE THIRD DILUTION OFTEN ACTS AS POWERFULLY AS A DRY GLOBULE. It also may explain the reason why Count Mattei insists that the remedies shall, as a rule, be taken in diluted forms.

8. That we are constantly meeting with evidence of the power of the infinitely little. The infinitely small and imponderable particles which float in the air and convey the sensation of smell have a great influence. The whole organism may be excited by them. Indeed it is said that the mere smell of prussic acid has sufficed to cause death. The smell of Russian leather in a room will prevent the fungi of mould from growing. The tiny bacilli of cholera, so small as to be hardly visible under a microscope magnifying [illegible]oo diameters, as well as the germs of consumption, small-pox or influenza, can slay the strong man armed.

9. That the susceptibility of a patient to the action of minute forces is immensely increased by disease. We sometimes lay straw down in the streets because he cannot bear the vibrations produced by the tiny waves of sound. We are often compelled to darken the windows of his room because he cannot tolerate the beating of the rays of light. Is it, then, a strange thing if he who is so susceptible to the action of agents which are external to him should be equally susceptible to the action of agents which are introduced into the channels through which his life-currents flow?

10. That the infinitely little has a strange power even upon the healthy subject. Professor Dundas has shown

that a solution of atropine in the proportion of 1 to 400,000 is sufficiently strong to completely dilate the pupil of the eye. Even the orthodox medical men have fixed the medicinal dose of sulphate of atropine at $\frac{1}{5000}$ of a grain. Rosenthal has shown that muscular fibre is extraordinarily sensitive to certain substances, that one part of these in from 1,000 to 2,000 parts of water affords strong contraction, and that the slightest amount of ammonia in tobacco smoke is sufficient to elicit continued pulsation.

11. Even upon organisms which are less sensitive than ours the infinitely little exerts a mighty influence. Darwin showed that $\frac{1}{20000000}$ of a grain exercised a visible action upon the leaves of the Drosera rotundi folia; Duelos found that plants watered with an aqueous solution of oxide of silver, in which the latter existed in the proportion of 1 to 1,000,000 stopped growing; and Gourbuyre discovered that fishes placed in twenty quarts of water in which a milligram of mercury had been dissolved soon ceased to live.

12. That Professor Crookes has taught that there are thousands of tons of energy stored up in every cubic inch of ether.

The objection to small doses is so common that we must be pardoned for lingering over this subject. If what has been already written does not suffice, we must ask the question which Mattei asks his readers: "What is the weight of the matter that the insect introduces with its poisonous sting and that causes men to die? Answer this, and then say whether you think it requires a larger quantity of matter to excite an equal and opposite reaction which shall bring to naught the deadly action of the poison." Those who plead for strong doses forget the power of little things. Facts like those just quoted should be remembered by our opponents.

Nor should they forget that if a small portion of virus has been introduced into the body it must have undergone considerable dilution ere it has penetrated the lowest layers of tissue, the minutest capillaries. Is it unreasonable to suppose that the remedy must be similarly diluted if it is to reach these places ?

EFFECTS OF THE REMEDIES.

The first effect of the remedies may be the production of a more hopeful spirit. Then there may follow various symptoms which are indicative of the expulsive powers of the medicines. For the poison which is in the system is frequently driven off through unusually abundant perspirations, slight eruptions or painless diarrhœa. Care must be taken not to suppress any of these as long as they are not too excessive. The general health gradually improves and at length the local affection subsides. When this happens patients are generally very anxious to discontinue the treatment, forgetting that no cure can be regarded as satisfactory which is not complete, and that sometimes when the outside of the vessel has been cleaned there are impurities lurking in its hidden recesses. It is highly important that the use of the chief remedies should be continued for some time after every symptom has disappeared. In cancer cases the use of *Scrofoloso giappone* and occasionally of *Canceroso*, should be continued to the end of life.

The length of time taken to effect a cure varies in different cases. Sometimes a single application of Electricity suffices. At other times weeks or months must elapse before the disease has been completely banished from the throne which it has usurped.

VII.—OTHER HYGIENIC HELPS.

HEALTH comes to those who keep the laws of nature rather than to those who defy them. Every health-seeker, therefore, should use ordinary hygienic measures as well as take curative remedies. Otherwise he may pull down by his carelessness the structure which he is attempting to build up by the remedies which he is taking. We cannot here recapitulate the laws of health which have been so clearly stated by numerous modern writers but must content ourselves with giving a few brief hints.

1. *Diet.*—Eat sufficient food but on no account take more than you require. It will do you less harm to eat too little than to take too much. Masticate your food. Do not bolt it. Remember that the saliva begins the work of digestion by transforming starch into sugar, and that much of this work should be done while the food is in the mouth. Do not eat or drink any food which is likely to cause discomfort on account of its excessive heat. If possible have a short rest before and twenty minutes rest after meals, especially after dinner. Take some ripe fruit at every meal. Grapes, apples, bananas, prunes, figs, and raisins are specially valuable in most cases. On account of the sugar which they contain, however, sufferers from skin affections, diabetes, &c., should avoid the two last. The delicate, the aged, and the convalescent should use only light but substantial food. Such articles as oatmeal porridge, wheat-

meal, barleymeal, &c., are specially valuable, because they are easily digested and highly nutritious. Some people, however, find oatmeal too heating. Sufferers from cutaneous diseases are specially liable to be unpleasantly affected by it. Anæmic patients require eggs, milk, well-cooked beef and mutton and other equally nutritious food. Patients who suffer from habitual costiveness should prefer a largely vegetarian diet. They should avoid much farinaceous food and should make a practice of taking fruit at every meal and particularly at breakfast. The custom of eating one or two bananas or apples before breakfast may be strongly commended. Dyspeptics should abstain from salt fish and meats, shell fish (except oysters) and all forms of pork and pastry. They should also avoid the excessive use of starchy foods, such as potatoes, white bread, tapioca, and arrowroot. When drinking milk they should be careful to take it in sips. In some cases it is a good practice to drink half-a-pint of warm water twenty minutes before each meal. Sufferers from skin eruptions should avoid greasy rich food and sweets and should use eggs, milk, cream and cheese very sparingly. They should eat green vegetables freely. Well-washed lettuces and water-cresses, if they can be well digested, are specially valuable in skin diseases.

2. *Dress*—Clothing has a great deal to do with health. Through carelessness with reference to this matter patients retard, if they do not altogether prevent their recovery. Every one should clothe lightly but warmly. The vital organs should be specially well protected from atmospheric changes, but no part of the body should be left insufficiently protected. Many childrens'

lives are lost simply because their parents take more pride in exhibiting the comeliness of their limbs than in keeping them from the freezing influences of wintry winds. All clothing which irritates or which prevents the free action of any part of the body is injurious. The lungs and heart should be allowed free play. Tight lacing is a proof of ignorance of what is healthful and beautiful, or of indifference to it. In skin diseases it is wise to avoid wearing flannel next the skin, as it often causes irritation and aggravates the ailment.

3. *Pure Air*—If the blood is the life of the body, oxygen is the life of the blood. Without oxygen the blood could not perform its functions and the man must die. Unless the proper proportion of oxygen is inhaled at each breath the physical mechanism suffers injury, and even the thinking powers grow less. Many a sleepy congregation yawns wearily, not because the preacher has insufficient interesting matter in his sermon, but because the church has insufficient oxygen in its atmosphere. Many a weary man wishes he had an extra hour in bed in the morning, not because he has spent insufficient time there already, but because the amount of poisonous gas in his bedroom has filled him with a deep sense of lethargy. It is a good rule to keep the door or window of sitting and bed rooms always open.

4. *Exercise* — Every part of the body should be properly exercised. The limb which is left unused will become atrophied. Exercise in the open air is specially valuable. Many a dyspeptic who is now a gloomy pessimist, would find the horizons of life becoming brighter if he spent two or three hours daily in open air exercise.

Many ladies who suffer from *ennui* would find life becoming suffused with a strange new light if they used artificial means of locomotion less, and natural means more. Thousands of anaemic school-girls owe their pallor chiefly to the fact that they spend too many hours over books which men have written, and too few in studying the great book of God which lies unrolled all around them.

5. *Cleanliness* — The regular use of baths and the practice of at least sponging the whole body over every day is highly important. Sufferers from skin diseases should use rain water or water which has been boiled and should avoid rough towels. They should also be careful not to use irritating soaps.

6. *Avoidance of Bad Habits.* — All excesses and hurtful practices should be shunned. Every medical man could write a startling exposition of the oft-quoted Bible text, "He that soweth to his own flesh shall of the flesh reap corruption." The man who seeks pleasure in ways that involve a breach of the highest laws will find that fleeting gratification has been followed by abiding misery. In many cases the stream of sorrow will flow on and deepen even to the third and fourth generation of his descendants. The wise man, therefore, will keep himself pure and sober. Strong passions of all kinds should be curbed. Jealousy, hate, grief, worry, are hurtful and should not be allowed to overcome us. Excessive smoking and the abuse of intoxicating liquors should be avoided. Indeed it is held by a growing number of the ablest physicians that the seeker after health had better leave the weed and the wine cup alone. Narcotics, such as opium and choral, should not be touched.

VIII.—HINTS TO BEGINNERS.

1. As a rule the patient may continue to take his ordinary diet, taking care, however, to AVOID ACIDS, especially lemons and vinegar.

2. The Electricities should be applied to the seat of pain as well as to the nerve-centres indicated below.

3. In applying the Red and Yellow Electricities for the relief of pain wait to see whether the former has sufficed before trying the latter.

4. But for simple tonic action on the nervous system the Electricities should be alternated in rapid succession.

5. Each remedy acts immediately. A dose of a second remedy may therefore follow without delay.

6. The dose should be increased as the disease yields to treatment, except in cases where massive doses have been used at the commencement to counteract previous drug treatment. In these instances it is only after the system becomes normally sensitive that the rule applies.

7. Interruption of treatment should be avoided. Otherwise relapses may follow. Care should be taken to avoid squandering the new strength begotten by the treatment.

8. Treatment should be continued for some time after the symptoms have disappeared, inasmuch as disease often lurks in hiding places after being expelled from the more prominent positions. Chronic cases of long standing

require warchful care during the second and third months of treatment. Premature exertion often makes it necessary to commence the treatment over again.

9. In desperate cases, after the ordinary treatment has failed, 40 to 50 globules of the remedy indicated may be dissolved in six ounces of water and given to the patient. Or 40 to 50 drops of *White* or *Blue* Electricity may be be given. Massive doses often compel the manifestation of deep-seated mischief. Half the disorders complained of are secondary, and it is essential to lay bare the root of the disease.

10. The administration of *Scrof. 1* or *5* or of *Angioitico 3* or *1* may often assist in diagnosing a case. If the disease is within the sphere of its operation the remedy will speedily produce amelioration. *Ang. 2* or *3* applied in a lotion, compress, or ointment over the part affected prepares the way for effective use of the proper Electricity or appropriate remedy.

11. It is not to be supposed that the remedies indicated in the following pages are to be given in a mechanical way nor that all are to be taken at once or successively.

12. It has already been stated that previous drug treatment may have made it necessary to adminster massive doses. When this is not the case the pint dilution for men, and the litre or quart for women and children, are best to start with, unless the symptoms shew that the patient is likely to be very sensitive to one or more of the various *groups of remedies*.

13. If any very marked effect followed the first few sips of the dilution given, it is well to reduce it to half the strength, and in all cases where the circulation is much

affected *Angioitico* should at first only be used in ointment, or at most in single dry globules, and afterwards the second dilution may be given sparingly.

14. Many persons desiring to use Count Mattei's remedies are wholly unaccustomed to the practice of Homœopathy and find it very difficult to believe in the efficacy of such minute doses, or that in cases of serious illness the dilutions must be *more attenuated.* Yet this is so, unless, indeed, the vital powers be *greatly exhausted*, and then, even a little child, may require stronger doses than will suffice for a powerful man under *ordinary conditions.*

15. The dose has to be nicely adjusted to each special case, and in order to do this anyone who wishes to become a *skilful* Matteist should seize opportunities of treating *slight* ailments of *various* kinds. Much may be learnt by practising on domestic animals, and the doses may often be given quite as strong as for a man.

16. It has been stated that persons who have been under ordinary drug treatment often require a course of dry globules (especially *Scrof. 5*) to render them normally sensitive to the Electro-Homœopathic remedies. Now it will be observed that dry globules are directed among the remedies enumerated for various disorders. As a rule it is best to make sure that the skin, lungs, kidneys, and bowels act well, under the influence of the dilutions, before giving dry globules, as the latter have a tonic action and sometimes may hinder the elimination of impurities from the system. On the other hand, in chronic cases, after the dilutions have been taken regularly for some time, it is often better to drop them by degrees and give dry globules.

17. The beginner is advised to use only White Electricity at first either applied on thick white blotting paper one inch square, or by gentle friction with the tips of three fingers. The Blue Electricity may next be tried and the Green for joint pains or sores of almost any kind. The Red and Yellow are best left to the last, and will be used most successfully by those who have first acquired some knowledge of the effects of the other three. In lymphatic ailments the Red and Yellow are of wonderful efficacy and in many cases will relieve pain at once. If any of the Electricities act too powerfully *Scrof. 1* should be given and a dose of 5, 7, or 10 globules will remove any discomfort.

18. When several remedies seem to be required at once it is best to select at least two for external use in ointments, liniments, or lotions.

19. Treatment should usually be begun with No. 1 of the Antiscrofoloso series or No. 3 of the Antiangioitic series. It should be borne in mind that *Scrofolosc* is useful in all kinds of inflammation, and *Angioitico* in all congestive disorders.

20. The more frequent the dose of the dilutions the smaller must be its amount.

21. The more frequent the dose of the dilutions the more rapid the cure, provided that the effects cause no discomfort. No remedy should be taken with such frequency or in such a potency as to produce any unpleasant sensations.

22. If no good effect follow the use of a remedy this proves that the dose is not suitable, that the wrong number of the group has been chosen, that the diagnosis has been

incorrect, and the wrong remedy applied, that the patient suffers from worms, ***which often cause failure***, or that the disease is incurable.

23. In the first case the dose should be altered from the second to the third or first dilution. The fiercer the disease, and the more sensitive the patient, the more must the remedy be diluted.

24. In the second case another number must be used. After trying *Scrof. 1* use *Scrof. 2* or *Scrof. 3.* After trying *Ang. 3* use *Ang. 2* or *Ang. 1.*

25. In the third case substitute a remedy belonging to another group, *i.e.*, an Antiangioitic for an Antiscrofulous or an Antilymphatic, and *vice versâ.*

26. If two or three remedies are used devote a part of each day to each, or better still, take them alternately throughout the day.

27. The dilutions are MOST IMPORTANT. The best results cannot be obtained without them.

28. If only one remedy is prescribed, a tumblerful should be taken in the course of the day in teaspoonful doses. If two remedies are prescribed, take either half-a-tumblerful of each, or three-quarters of a tumblerful of the one which is most needed, and a quarter of a tumblerful of the other. In some cases, however, only a few teaspoonfuls a day can be taken with benefit. In acute cases (fevers, &c.) it is sometimes necessary to give very small doses every 5 minutes. In other cases sips should be taken frequently, so that the whole quantity prescribed is used in the course of the day. Persevere with these. As a rule begin treatment with the intermediate, second or third dilution. Afterwards it is often advisable to go

on to the first dilution.

29. The globules prescribed for use in beverage at meals may be taken at three or four meals from three to five globules at a time. If two kinds are prescribed use them alternately.

30. The Electricities should usually be applied to the places numbered in the diagram 5, 6, 17, 18 and also to any group of nerves directly affected by the disease. If two Electricities are prescribed the second should be used after a few seconds' interval. They should be applied once, twice or thrice daily.

31. Sometimes more remedies are named than are needed in any one case. The patient should first try the first one or two mentioned. If these fail to benefit him let him use some of the others. Experience will teach him how to select those best suited to his case.

Count Mattei has been so deeply impressed with the teachings of Doctors Charazain and Dècle with reference to the polarity of the body, that he has introduced them into his books. Many Matteists have grave doubts respecting their accuracy. Others declare that the best effects follow the use of the positive and negative Electricities in harmony with the laws of polarity stated by these doctors, according to whom :

1. The right half of the face and neck are negative.
2. The left half of the face and neck are positive.
3. The outer side of the arms and legs are positive.
4. The inner side of the arms and legs are negative.
5. The right half of the chest and back are negative.
6. The left half of the chest and back are positive.
7. The parts on a line drawn along the centre of the

human body from the centre of the skull, before and behind, are both positive and negative.

As the healer aims at the restoration of the normal condition, Count Mattei has taught his disciples to apply the contrary Electricities to the positive and negative parts.

ABBREVIATIONS USED IN THE TABLES.

A or Ang.—Antiangioitico or Angioitico (remedy for the angioitic or over-sanguine state).

Alt.—Alternated with.

B. or B. El.—Blue Electricity (specially for angioitic patients, braces the nerves and veins and checks hæmorrhage.)

C. or Canc.—Canceroso, or Anticanceroso (for tumours, cancers, &c.

Comp.—Compress.

Dil.—Dilution.

E.—Evening.

F. or Feb.—Febrifugo, or Febrifuge (specific for fevers, also useful in disorders of the liver, spleen, &c.)

G. or G. El.—Green Electricity (a powerful pain-killer, especially in cancer cases and in articular rheumatism.

Garg.—Gargle.

Glob.—Globules (i.e., little pills.)

Inj.—Injections.

L. or Lin.—Linfatico.

Lit.—Litre (1⅞ pints.)

Ly.—Lymphatic temperament.

Mi.—Mixed temperament.

M.—Morning.

Oint.—Ointment.

P. or Pet.—Pettorale (pectoral for coughs, colds, &c.)

R. or R. El.—Red Electricity (excites the nerves and quickens the circulation.)

S. or Scrof.—Scrofoloso or Antiscrofoloso (remedy for scrofulous and allied conditions.)

Sg. or Scrof. Giap.—Scrofoloso Giappone.

Sa.—Sanguine or angioitic temperament.

Ven.—Anti-venereo or Venereo (for the worst form of constitutional taint.)

Ver.—Vermifugo (a remedy for worms.)

W. or W. El.—White Electricity (useful as a nerve tonic.)

Y. or Y. El.—Yellow Electricity (relaxes nerve tension and restores too rapid circulation to its normal rate. A useful laxative and vermifuge.)

FIGURES.

The figure following the name of the remedy indicates which remedy in the particular group bearing the name is to be used. Thus *Canc. 5* the fifth of the Canceroso series of remedies. When referring to the first of the series the number is often left out. Thus *Canc.*—the first of the Canceroso group.

The numerals used to indicate parts to which Compresses, Ointments, or Electricities should be applied are the following:

1. *Super-orbital*: The nerve-point above the eye.

2. *Sub-orbital*: The nerve-point below the eye.

3. *Base of Nose.*

4. *Brachial*: The principal points at which the chief nerve controlling the arm come to the surface.

5. *Solar-plexus*: A most important ganglion of nerves which exerts so powerful an influence over the body that Stahl assigned to it the seat of the soul, and Van Helmont regarded it as the centre of vitality.

6. *Pit of Stomach*: The solar plexus extends over this part.

7. *Gastric Sympathetic*: The portion of the sympathetic nerve distributed over the stomach.

8. *Crural*: The main nerve of the front of the leg.

9. *Small Hypoglossi*: Nerves which originate in the back of the head and are connected with the great hypoglossi.

10. *Small muscles behind the ear*: Apply positive electricity on the right side and negative on the left.

11. *Occiput*: The occipital nerve at the nape of the neck.

12. *Cervical Sympathetic*: Ganglia on both sides of the spine. Positive Electricity should be applied to the one on the right hand. Negative Electricity should be applied to the other.

13. *Great Hypoglossi*: Nerves whose branches are distributed to the under surface of the tongue.

14. *Sciatic Nerve*: A nerve extending from the sacral

nerves along the back of the leg. It comes near the surface at the points marked 14 in the diagram.

15. *Arch of the foot.*

16. *Small Hypoglossi* (See 9.)

17. *Occiput* (See 11.)

18. *Sympathetic*: The nerves situated above and below the 7th vertebra and connecting the ganglia numbered 12. The sympathetic nerve controls the circulation. To increase the speed of the circulation the sympathetic nerve should be stimulated by application of *Blue* or *Red* Electricity. To diminish the speed of the circulation *Yellow* Electricity should be applied.

19. *Bottom of Stomach.*

20. *Sacral nerves*, which branch out from both sides of the lower end of the spine.

21. *Loins.*

22. *Perineum* : The part in front of the anus.

23. *Forehead.*

24. *Hypochondriac region* : The part (shaded in the diagram) in which the liver and spleen are situated.

25. *Pubes* : The part of the body behind which the bladder is situated.

26. *Dorsal Spine* : The middle part of the spine.

27. *Heart.*

28. *Pneumogastric Nerve* : To diminish the speed of circulation, the pneumogastric nerve should be stimulated by applications of *Blue* or *Red* El. To increase the speed of the circulation *Yellow* El. should be applied.

29. *Ovaries* : (In women).

INCUBATIVE PERIODS.

There are many cases in which it is useful to know the length of time which elapses between the entrance of a disease germ into the system and the appearance of the first symptoms of its victory. The following will, therefore, be valuable:

Cholera	From a few hours to four days.
Dengue	3 days.
Diphtheria	3 days to 8 days.
Influenza	A few hours.
Malaria	10 to 12 days.
Measles	10 days to the sickening, 12 days to the rash.
Mumps	10 to 21 days.
Pertussis	4 days to 14 days.
Plague	1 to 5 days.
Rabies	14 days to many months.
Relapsing Fever	5 days.
Röthlein	10 to 21 days.
ScarletFever ...	2 to 7 days.
Small-pox	12 days to illness, 14 days to eruption.
Syphilis	10 days to induration, rash or sore throat six weeks later.
Yellow Feevr...	2 to six days.

THE REMEDIES FOR VARIOUS DISEASES.

Abscess. A collection of pus in a superficial or deep-seated part of the body. This pus is formed of albumen which has exuded through the capillaries in consequence of their being overcharged with blood through inflammation. The several varieties of abscess require different treatment:

1. *Cold Abscess* occurs generally in lymphatic subjects; developes slowly and painlessly. The pus in this is generally very watery. Take *Scrof. 1* or *2*, first dil. or *Scrof. 5*, first dil. while it is closed, and use *Canc. 1* or *Canc. 5* Ointment. When it suppurates take 5 globs. *Scrof. 1* or *Scrof. 5* dry on the tongue every morning, and 5 globs. *Scrof. 1* or *Canc. 5* dry on the tongue in the evening and in beverage at meals. During the day take *Canc. 1*, first dil. or Canc. 4, first dil. Baths of *Canc. 5* and ointments or compresses of *Canc. 5* or *Canc. 1* alt. *Scrof. 5* may also be used. Apply *Red* and *Yellow* El. to 17, 18, 5, and to nerves corresponding with the part in which the abscess is located. In obstinate cases use dilutions of *Ang. 1* alt *Canc. 1*. Compresses, ointments and baths of *Ang. 3* alt. *Canc. 1* or *Canc. 5*. Apply *White* El.

2. *Acute Inflammatory Abscess* with throbbing pain, bright redness before suppuration begins and livid skin

with less pain after it commences; constitutional disturbance with chilliness. Fever and thirst are marked, especially when the abscess is deep seated. The pus is thick and of a greenish yellow colour. Morning and evening: 5 globs. *Scrof. 1* dry; *Ang. 1* second dil. alt. *Canc. 1*, first dil. with frequent teaspoonfuls of *Feb. 1*, second or third dil.; if there is much pus one globule *Canc. 5* hourly, dry. Compresses *Canc. 5* alt. *Ang. 3* to the abscess with *Feb. 2* (10 globules) to 24. Baths *Canc. 5* and *Scrof. 5*. *Red* and *Yellow* El. to the principal nerve centres; *Ang. 3* ointment to 27; *Feb. 2* ointment to 24; 5 drops *Blue* El. on cranium. Abscess in the breast requires at first *Canc. 1*, first dil. with 5 globs. *Scrof.* night and morning, and afterwards *Canc.* second dil., alt. *Scrof.* second dil., with *Canc. 5* ointment around it.

3. *Chronic Congestive Abscess*, with serous pus, resulting from disease of the bone: *Canc. 1* first or second dil., alt. sometimes with *Ang. 1* litre dil.; *Canc. 1* at meals; 1 glob. *Canc. 1* hourly. Compress *Canc. 4* or *Canc. 5*. Should this treatment not suffice try *Canc. 4*, *Canc. 5*, or *Lin.* in dil. *Red* and *Yellow* El. Baths, *Canc. 5*, *Scrof. 5*; ointment *Feb. 2*, to 24.

4. *Syphilitic Abscesses* require *Ven.*

Accidents. See Bruises, &c.

Accouchement. To facilitate, use *Scrof. 1* dil. during pregnancy; injections of *Canc. 5* (15 globules in a half-pint of water), and weekly baths of *Canc. 5* (50 globules). At the time of labour take 4 *Canc. 1* dry every half hour, or take *Canc. 1* in second dil.

Acidity. (See also Indigestion). *Scrof. 1* litre or second dil., or *Canc. 1* second dil. (In graver cases alternated with *Ang. 1* second dil.) Apply *Red* El. to 6 twice a day; *Feb. 2* ointment to 24, or *Feb. 1* litre dil. if *Scrof. 1* fails to relieve.

Acne. Isolated, pointed pustules or pimples, caused by congestion of the sebaceous follicles. There are several varieties. *Acne punctata* (maggot-pimple), from which a small maggot-like piece of matter may be squeezed out; *acne indurata* (stone-pock), hard pimples producing a sense of tightness in the face; *acne rosacea* (rosy-drop), caused by drinking alcohol, but sometimes occuring in women whose periodical functions are disturbed, and in plethoric and other persons. *Scrof.* second dil. alt. *Canc.* Lotions of *Canc. 5* and *Acqua-per-la-pelle.* Compresses, *Canc. 5.* Baths of *Canc. 5* alt. *Scrof. 1* or *Scrof. 5.* Sanguine patients, however, should use *Ang.* second dil., and baths of *Ang. 3* instead of those of *Canc. 5* or *Scrof.*

In *Syphilitic acne* use litre dil. *Ven.* or *Ven.* alt. *Canc. 5.*

Addison's Disease. An obscure and little understood disease of the supra-renal capsules (obscure glands situated above the kidneys), accompanied by a peculiar discolouration or bronzing of the skin, increasing muscular debility, and marked anæmia. Try *Canc. 1* litre dil., 1 glob. *Canc. 5* hourly. 3 to 5 globs. *Scrof. 1* at meals. Baths of *Canc. 5* alt. *Scrof. 5. Lin.* ointment across loins, and *Ang. 3* ointment to heart. *Red* El. to 20 and six points. 2 dry globs. *Lin.* every morning.

Adenitis: Congestion or acute inflammation of the absorbent glands, with pain and in many cases feverishness.

1. *Acute Congestion.* *Scrof. 1* first dil. or *Scrof. 1* alt. *Ang.* second dil. with *Feb. 1* second dil. if there is feverishness. Compress of *Red* El. and *Scrof.* to 20. When the throbbing heat and inflammation show that suppuration is about to commence take *Scrof. 1* alt. *Canc. 1* first dil., and use compress of *Canc. 5* to 20. When suppuration has set in, use *Canc. 5* ointment around abscess instead of compress. After it has ended take *Scrof. 1* first dil., and use compresses of *Scrof. 1* to 20 and *Blue* El. Baths of *Canc. 5* alt. *Ang. 1* or *Ang. 3.* *Red* and *Yellow* El. to related nerves.

2. *Chronic Congestion.* *Scrof 1* first or second dil., or *Scrof. 2* alt. *Canc. 1*, always in the first dil. (to promote suppuration, the second and third dil. of *Canc. 1* would retard it). Only 10 teaspoonfuls of these dilutions should be taken daily. Should small tumours form around the inflamed gland, use *Lin.* or *Scrof. 5* ointment to them. Should suppuration not proceed satisfactorily take 10 globs. *Canc. 5* morning and evening, dry. In obstinate cases use baths of *Scrof. 5* alt. *Canc. 5* alt. *Ang. 3.* Compresses *Green* El. After a cure has been effected continue using *Scrof. 1* for some months. Pure air, good food, and ample exercise, &c., are of great importance in this complaint.

After Pains relieved by *Canc. 1*, first dil.

Ague. See Intermittent Fever.

Alba Dolens Plegmasia. See White Leg.

Albino (Lincopathy) a disease to which negroes are most subjected, consisting in the absence of the colouring matter beneath the cuticle and the true skin. Treated by application of Compresses of *White* El. to head and of *Red* or *Red* El. alt. *Yel.* El. to 12, 18, 2, 3, forehead. Ointment of *Can. 5* alt. *Scrof. 1* alt. *Ang. 2.*

Albugo. *Scrof. 1* second dil. or *Canc. 1* second dil. alt. *Ang. 1* second dil. in grave cases.

Albuminuria, a disease occurring either together with Bright's disease or independently of it, and which is characterised by an injurious waste of albumen through the urinary organs. *Scrof. 1* first dil., or *Lin.* with Compresses of *Scrof. 1* or *Scrof. 5* to the kidneys. *Red* El. to kidneys. Baths *Canc. 5* or *Scrof 5* alt. *Ang. 2.* Ointment *Scrof. 5* or *Lin.* to kidneys. Should this fail to lessen the loss, take *Scrof. 1* second dil. alt. *Ang. 2* second dil. and 5 *Scrof. 1* dry on the tongue night and morning. Also 1 *Canc. 5* hourly. If there is any feverishness use *Feb. 1* second or third dil. and *Feb. 2* ointment to 24.

Alcoholism. The drunkard cannot hope for cure unless he becomes a total abstainer. Should he do this he may gradually obtain deliverance from his craving by *Ang. 1* second dil. or by *Ang. 1*, first or second dil. alt. *Scrof. 1*, third dil.

Alopœcia. Baldness of head or falling off of beard, following debilitating illness. *Scrof. 1*, first dil. *Scrof. 5* and *Canc. 5* ointments. Alcoholised lotion of *Scrof. 5* or *Lin.* When the hair or beard comes off in round patches *Ven.* also must be used in dilution and compresses.

Amaurosis. Blindness caused by disease of the optic nerve. Some of its forms are curable by means of *Scrof.* *Scrof. 2* or *Canc.* second dil. when the origin is nervous, with compresses of *White* El. to the head and the application of *Red* or of *Red* alt. *Yel.* El. to the corresponding nerves (17, 18, 2, 3, and forehead.)

Anæmia (Poverty of Blood): A disease of which females from 15 to 25 years of age are most frequently the subjects. The patients are pale and bloodless, waxy-looking or greenish. They suffer from cold extremities, irritability, and neuralgic and hysterical pains in different parts of the body. Menstruation is usually deranged. Leucorrhœa often accompanies anæmia. The Mattei remedies have been exceptionally useful in these cases. Lymphatic patients require *Scrof. 1* first dil., and at meals (6 glob. twice daily) dry glob. of *Lin.* Baths of *Lin.* alt. *Ang. 3.* Apply *Red* and *Yel.* El. to 5, 6, 17, 18. Angioitic patients: *Ang.* alt. *Lin.* or *Scrof.* If puffy, *Ang. 2.* Same at meals. Baths *Ang 3.* Ointment of *Ang. 2* or *3* to heart. Those who suffer also from Leucorrhœa need *Ang. 1* alt. *Canc. 1*, second dil.; 1 glob. *Canc. 5* hourly. Baths of *Ang. 2* or *3* alt. *Canc. 5.* Ointment of *Feb. 2* to 24. Injections of *Canc. 1* or *5* alt. *Ang. 3.* Cheerful society, bracing air, and nutritious food are helpful.

Analgesia: absence of pain, want of sensitiveness. *Canc. 1*, second dil. alt. *Ang 1*, second dil. Glycerine and spirit liniment of *Ang. 2.* *Scrof. 5* dry, also *Scrof. 5* ointment.

Anaphrodisia. Sexual impotence, *Scrof. 1*, litre or second dil. or *Canc. 1*, second dil. Some cases also require *Ang. 1*, second dil. Baths of *Canc. 1*, *Scrof. 1.*

Anasarca: See Dropsy. *Scrof. 2* and *Canc. 2* litre dil., and *Ang. 2* second dil.

Anchylosis (Ankylosis): Stiffness of any joint. Usually the result of disease. *Scrof. 1* or *Scrof. 2* dil. alt. *Lin.* Compress of *Canc. 1.* *Red* and *Yel.* El. to 5, 6, 17,

18, 19. Baths of *Lin.*, *Canc. 5*, *Scrof. 5*, *White* El. Should these remedies fail try *Canc. 5*, *Canc. 2*, or *Canc. 4* alt. *Ang. 1*, second dil. and compress of *Blue* or *Green* El.

Aneurism: A tumour formed by the dilatation of the walls of an artery. Moisten the hand with a few drops of *Blue* El. and pass lightly over the heart. Compresses of *Ang. 3* or *2*. *Ang. 3* or *1* second or third dil., 5 to 8 teaspoonfuls daily.

Angina: Constriction of the throat or chest with inflammation of the mucous membrane.

1. *Guttural angina* is characterised by feverishness, pain, and redness in the throat, with the secretion of a thready mucus, swollen and elongated uvula. For the Fever *Feb. 1*, a teaspoonful every 5 or 10 minutes. *Scrof.* second dil. or *Canc.* second dil. alt. *Ang. 1*, second dil. Apply *Red* alt. *Yel.* El. to 5, 6, 7, 17, 18. Gargles of *Red* or *Blue* El. Ointments *Canc. 5* alt. *Ang. 3* to the whole of the throat and back of the neck, and *Ang. 3* to the heart. If obstinate try *Canc. 1* or *Canc 4* or *Canc. 1* alt. *Canc. 4* and *Dom Fin*, second dil. *Dom Fin* ointment. If there is cough add *Pet.* litre dil.

2. *Angina Pectoris* (Breast pang). An obscure affection probably of the nerves belonging to the cardiac plexus. Generally sets in suddenly with intense pain or even excruciating torture in the neighbourhood of the heart, a feeling of constriction across the chest and a sense of suffocation. Followed by pallid face covered with cold sweat. *Scrof.* or *Canc.* alt. *Pet.* Ointment *Canc. 5* over chest, and warm compress of *Ang. 2* to heart. Gargles *Red* El. *Canc. 5.* Avoid indigestible food. Tone up the system by nourishing and unstimulating diet, fresh air, &c.

3. *Pseudo-membranous*: Sharp pain in throat accompanying formation of false grey membrane. *Scrof.* or *Canc.* second dil. alt. *Ang. 1*, second dil. 1 glob. *Canc. 5* dry hourly. Gargles of *Canc. 5 Red* or *White* El. Ointment *Ang. 2* to heart, *Feb. 2* to hypochondria, *Canc. 5* and *Ang. 2* to throat. *Red* alt. *Yel.* to related nerves.

Angioitis. Inflammation of the vascular system accompanied by erysipelas, eruptions, &c. *Ang. 1* or *Ang. 2* second dil., alt. *Canc. 5* second dil. Baths, *Canc. 5* alt. *Ang. 3.*

Anorexia. Loss of appetite, sometimes amounting to disgust with food. *Scrof.* second dil. or *Canc.* second dil., alt. *Ang.* second dil. in grave cases. 3 globs. *Scrof.* (dry) every morning. *Red* El. alt. *Yellow* El. to 6. Baths, *Canc. 5* alt. *Lin.*

Anthrax. Boil-like swellings in various parts of the cellular tissue, with feverishness and nausea. *Feb. 1* second dil., afterwards *Scrof.* 1 glob. *Canc. 5* hourly. Same treatment as in Carbuncle.

Anus: Condylomata Ani. Warty excrescences of a syphilitic character. *Ven.* alt. *Canc. 4*, second dil. Compress *White* El. alt. *Canc 1* alt. *Canc. 5.* Application of *Red* alt. *Yel.* to perineum and down the spine. Baths of *Canc. 5* alt. *Ven.* During convalescence use *Scrof. 1.*

Aphthæ. See Thrush.

Apparent Death. A few globules of *Scrof. 1* on the tongue.

Appetite, Loss of. See Anorexia.

Arm, Atrophy of. *Scrof.* dil. 3 globs. *Scrof.* dry morning. Compress, *White* El.; Apply *Red* El. alt.

Yellow El. to 17, 18, 5, 4. Baths of *Canc. 5* alt. *Scrof.* alt. *Ang. 3*, with ointments of the same.

Arm, Numbness in. Same treatment, with *Ang.* dil. in addition.

Arm, Semi-Anchylosis. Same treatment as in Atrophy of Arm.

Arthritis. An inflammation of the joints, with feverishness, which sometimes brings about great deformity. In the chronic variety one joint after another is rendered rigid, motionless, and either permanently bent or enlarged. 5 globs. *Scrof.* dry on tongue in morning; *Scrof.* or *Canc.* dil. (alt. *Ang.* in grave cases). Compresses, *Canc. 5* to hypochondriac region and *Ang. 3* to heart. Ointment of *Feb. 2* to hypochondria. Baths *Canc. 5* alt. *Scrof. 1.*

Aphonia. See loss of voice.

Apoplexy: Hæmorrhage within the cranium followed by sudden loss of consciousness. Usually preceded by sense of heaviness, vertigo, impaired memory, local twitchings. An attack is sometimes ushered in with a convulsion. The patient becomes comatose, the face often livid, and the breathing stertorous. Motor paralysis occurs on the side opposite to that on which the cerebral lesion has occurred.

1. *Sanguineous*: 8 to 20 globules *Scrof.* dry on tongue. Repeat every ten minutes till consciousness is restored. *Ang. 1* third dil., half-teaspoonful doses. *Blue* El. to heart and chief points. Compresses *Ang. 1* or *Ang. 2.* Apply *White* El. to seat of effusion.

2. *Serous*: Eight to 20 globules *Scrof. 1* dry on tongue. Repeat this dose every ten minutes while vomiting lasts, or until consciousness is restored, and

8

apply the Electricities to all the main points. *Scrof. 1* second or third dil., sometimes alt. with *Ang. 1* second dil. Remove all superfluous clothing. With *Hemiplegia*, add *Canc.* or *Scrof.* dil.; application of *Red* and *Yellow* El. to six points. Baths of *Scrof.* alt. *Ang. 3* alt. *Canc. 5.*

Ascites: Dropsy of the peritoneum. Skin generally appears stretched, thin and shining. The abdomen is enlarged. On change of position the fluid may be sometimes seen moving and the form of the abdomen undergoes modification. *Scrof.* second dil. alt. *Canc. 2*, second dil., with *Red* alt. *Yellow* El. to 17, 18. If the disease originate from the liver take *Feb.*, third dil. alt. *Canc. 2*, second dil. and ointment of *Feb. 2* to the liver. If from the heart *Ang. (1, 2, or 3,)* third dil. alt. *Canc. 2*, second dil., with gentle frictions of *Blue* El. to the heart (4 drops on palm of hand). It may be well to use the *Blue* El. alone sparingly, and then give the *Ang.* in third dil. after a few applications have been made.

Asphyxia: a cessation of pulsation with suspended respiration, arising from drowning, choking, &c. *Scrof.* or 10 to 20 globs. *Scrof.* all at once on the tongue. Apply *Red* alt. *Yellow* El. to 17, 18, 5, also to nape. *White* El. to cranium. Warm baths of *Canc. 5.* Unction of *Canc. 5* to 6, and all over head. *Ang. 2* ointment to heart.

Asthma: A disease characterised by habitual or spasmodic difficulty in breathing, accompanied by wheezing and tightness in the chest. Spasmodic attacks generally occur between two and four a.m., and are specially bad if the patient has taken a heavy supper, or inhales irritating gases or vapours, &c. There are several forms of Asthma.

1. *Bronchial*, sometimes results from a paralytic con-

dition of the bronchial tubes, but is generally due to spasm of the muscular fibres, excited through the nerves in consequence of mechanical or reflex irritation. Sometimes it arises from Cardiac disease. *Scrof. 1* second or third dil. or *Lin.* second dil. Apply *Red* El. to 6, 17, 18 or *Blue* if a heart affection is the cause of the trouble. In the latter case *Ang. 2* first or second dil. may be used alone, six doses daily, with 2 drops *Blue* El. every half hour. Also apply *Blue* El. to 27. When Asthma is associated with Bronchitis or bronchial irritation *Pet. 1* dil. must be alternated with the preceding. In all cases baths of *Canc. 5* and unction of *Canc. 5* to 18 are useful. In persons subject to Gout, Scrofula, Erysipelas, &c., asthmatic attacks may often be cut short by taking 5 to 8 dry globules of *Scrof. 1*, while sanguine patients may frequently obtain relief by taking 4 to 5 drops of *Blue* El. on a lump of sugar.

2. *Cardiac*: Panting or noisy breathing resulting from congestion of the venous system, associated with heart disease. *Ang. 1* second or third dil. and 4 teaspoonfuls of *Scrof. 1* third dil. per day. Gently apply *Blue* El. to heart (4 drops on palm of hand.)

3. *Congestive Asthma*, preceding monthly periods, requires *Ang. 1*, and *Blue* El. to heart.

Atrophy: Waste of tissue resulting from deficient nutrition, either general or local. Often accompanied by degeneration. *Scrof.* alt *Canc. 5* dil. and sometimes *Ang. 2.* Baths of *Scrof. 1* alt. *Canc. 5* alt. *Ang. 3*, or of *White* El. Applications of *Red* El. alt. *Yellow* El. alt. *Blue* El. to 18, 17, 5, and nerves of the parts affected. Ointment of *Feb. 2* and *Canc. 5* to the hypochondriac region.

Balanitis: Inflammation of the prepuce. *Scrof.* second dil. or *Canc.* second dil. if there is any ulceration or suppuration. Sitz baths of *Scrof. 1* or *Canc. 1* alt. *Ang. 3.*

Baldness: *Scrof. 1*, first dil. Ointment and lotion of *Scrof. 5.* See Alopœcia.

Beard, Loss of: *Scrof.* first dil. alt. *Canc.* second dil. Lotion of *Scrof. 5.* Ointment of *Scrof. 5* and *Canc.* If falling off in round patches, as a result of syphilis, *Ven.* in litre dil. is also required, with baths and ointments of *Canc. 5* and *Scrof. 1*, and *Ven.* ointment. *White* El.

Bilious attack: see Liver disorders.

Bites: *Dogs*: The wound should be cauterised and a Russian or vapour bath should be taken without delay. 20 globs. *Scrof.* should be taken dry and afterwards *Scrof. 1* dil. may be used with *Red* alt. *Yellow* El. to 12, 18, 5, 6. *Insects*: Compress of *Canc. 5*, or of *Blue* El. if there is much inflammation. Sometimes compress of *Red* or *White* El. *Lin.* or *Scrof.* is useful. 1 glob. *Canc. 5* hourly. Baths of *Scrof. 2, Ang. 2, Canc. 5.*

Bleeding: See Hæmorrhage.

Blenorrhagia: When this is syphilitic it is treated with *Ven.* litre dil., alt. *Scrof.* litre dil. or *Canc. 5* first dil. Injections of *Scrof.* or *Canc. 1* alt. *Canc 5.* When blood is present in the discharge, take 5 globs. *Canc.* night and morning, and *Ven.* first dil. alt. *Ang.* litre dil. during the day. The *Canc. 5* in dil. and *Canc. 1* injection should take the place of *Scrof.* when the discharge becomes greenish and there is great inflammation. When this happens 3 globs. *Scrof.* should be taken dry night and morning. For further hints see treatment for syphilis. When it is rheumatic it requires *Scrof. 1*, third dil., or *Scrof. 5*, third dil. alt. *Ang. 2*, second dil., if the circulation is defective.

Blenorrhœa: Military Gout: Treated with *Canc. 1*, litre dil. alt. *Ven.* litre dil., succeeded by *Canc. 2*, *Canc. 5*, and *Lin.* if the first fail. Injections of *Canc. 5*.

Blepharitis: Inflammation of the Eyelids. See Eyelids.

Blindness: See Eyes.

Blood Poisoning: See Pyæmia and Septicæmia.

Blood, Deficiency of, with sanguine stagnation, anæmia, chlorosis (green sickness), palpitation, slow pulse: *Ang. 1*, second or third dil., *Ang. 2*, second or third dil., or *Ang. 3*, second or third dil., with *Canc. 1*, second dil.

Bladder, Acute inflammation of the (Cystitis), caused by irritation, &c. Its presence is indicated by constant inclination to urinate, a difficulty in retaining urine, and pain in passing it. The urine is often red and burning. There are mucus in urine, tenderness, dull pain in the lower part of the abdomen, increased by pressure and by straining at stool. The passage of a whitish substance is a symptom of catarrh of the bladder. *Scrof. 6*, first dil., or *Scrof. 1*, second dil., with *Ang. 2*, second dil., in sanguine patients, and if there is blood in the urine, also 3 globs. *Feb. 1* dry morning and evening, or *Feb. 2* oint. Lotions of *Scrof. 1* and *Red* El. In obstinate cases *Canc. 1*. Compress of *White* El. to 20, 22, 25. Application of *Red* and *Yellow* El. to 5, 17, 18, 20, and loins. Warm baths of *Canc. 5* alt. *Scrof.* alt. *Ang. 3*, and ointments of *Canc. 5* alt. *Scrof.* applied locally with *Ang. 3* to the pubes and heart and *Feb. 2* to 24.

Chronic Catarrh of the, indicated by the presence of much epithelium and mucus in the urine. Same treatment except that second or third dil. of *Scrof. 6* should be used instead of the first. Warm baths and local fomentations, the water being medicated with *Canc. 5*, or *Lin.* alt. *Scrof.* alt. *Ang. 3.* Warm injections of *Scrof. 6* or *White* El. are sometimes useful.

Distention of the. Same treatment.

Paralysis of the. Same treatment and also injections of *White* El.

Polypus of the: see Polypus. *Canc. 4* and *Canc. 5* dil. with the remedies used for catarrh of the bladder.

Blood, Excess of, with congestion of the brain, lungs, &c. Treated with *Ang. 1*, second or third dil., *Ang. 2*, second or third dil., or *Ang. 3* second or third dil. with compresses of *Ang. 1* or *2*, [2 globules to a tablespoonful of water] over the heart, or gentle frictions of *Blue* El.

Blood, Spitting of. See Hæmoptysis.

Blood, Vomiting of. See Hæmatemesis.

Blows: Small compresses of *Red* or *Blue* El., covered with large compresses of *Scrof. 1* or *Scrof. 3.*

Blue Disease (Cyanosis). *Scrof. 3* alt. *Ang. 3*, a few teaspoonfuls of each daily.

Boils. See also Abscesses. To correct tendency to, *Scrof. 5* lit. dil. alt. *Ang. 1*, lit. dil. A small plaster over which *Canc. 5* ointment has been spread should be put on the boil. Or use compress of *Canc. 5* or *Scrof. 5* alt. *Ang. 3* if there is much inflammation. Apply *Red* and *Yellow* El. to 17, 18.

Bones, Abscess in. (See Abscess). (1.) *Anchylosis of Joint: Canc.* alt. *Ang.* dil. Lotions and ointments of *Canc.* alt. *Ang.* or *Scrof. 5* alt. *Lin.* (2.) *Caries of:* 3 globs. *Canc. 1* morning and 3 globs. *Canc. 5* night; *Canc. 4* first dil. or *Lin.*; 4 or 5 globs. *Scrof. 1* in beverage at meals. (3.) *Exostosis:* Swelling of the bone arising from Cancerous, Scrofulous, or Syphilitic virus. *Scrof.* or *Lin.* alt. *Canc. 4* or *Canc. 3* dil. Same remedies at meals. Lotions of *Scrof.* Baths of *Canc. 5.* Applications of *Blue* El. to sympathetic nerves. Compresses *Canc. 5* or *Canc. 4.* Ointment *Feb. 2* to 24. If Syphilitic, alternate *Ven.* with *Canc. 4* in dil. (4.) *Nodes:* Tumours on the surface of a bone, generally following Scrofulous or Syphilitic disease, accompanied by violent pains. *Scrof.* alt. *Canc. 3* alt. *Ang.* dil. Should this fail try also *Canc. 5.* Take 3 globs. *Canc. 4* dry night and morning. Ointment of *Canc. 5* alt. *Scrof.* or *Scrof. 5.* Compresses of *Ven.* alt. *Canc. 5* or *Scrof. 5*, *Scrof. 1*, *Canc. 4*; also compresses of *White* or *Red* El. Baths of *Canc. 5*, *Scrof. 1*, *Scrof. 5.* (5.) *Necrosis:* The death of the whole or part of a bone. *Canc. 3* or *Canc. 4*, dil. If Syphilitic origin is suspected *Ven.* third dil. alt. *Canc. 3* or *Canc. 4*, third dil. Compress with same remedies in diseased parts. *Canc. 5* ointment to the dorsal region of the spine. (6.) *Pains in:* Nocturnal, generally resulting from a more or less remote Syphilitic taint. *Scrof. 1* alt. *Ven.* alt. *Feb. 1* either dry or in dil. Compresses and ointments of *Scrof.* and *Blue* El. (7.) *Periostitis:* Inflammation of the periosteum. Same treatment as for Exostosis. (8.) *Spina Ventosa:* Dilation of the bone tissues, as if blown up by wind, with sharp piercing pains. *Canc. 4* second dil. alt. *Ang.* second dil., 5 globs.

Scrof. at meals. Baths of *Canc. 5.* Compresses of *Green* or *Red* alt. *Yellow* El.

Bowels: *Colic:* Sharp, griping pains, attended by irregular spasmodic contraction of the muscular coat of the intestines, resulting from direct or reflex irritation, morbid condition of the blood, &c. *Scrof.* or *Scrof. Giap.* first dil. half a teaspoonful every five minutes while the attack lasts; 1 glob. *Scrof.* dry every half hour. Apply *Red* alt. *Yellow* El. to 6, and *Canc. 5* ointment over abdomen. (1.) *Consumption of:* (See Tabes Mesenterica). (2.) *Inflammation of:* There are several varieties. Of these the simplest is enteric catarrh, due to irritation. This sometimes becomes chronic. It is characterised by uneasiness, gripy pains, rumbling noises in the intestines, and diarrhœa. Sometimes the tongue is red and furred and there is nausea. When the duodenum is involved there is sometimes some jaundice and pains in the back of the head. *Scrof.* second dil. alt. *Feb. 1*, or *Canc.* second dil. alt. *Scrof. Giap.* Baths of *Canc. 5.* Compress, *White* El. to abdomen. Unction, *Canc. 5* to abdomen. *Red* alt. *Yellow* El. to 18. (3.) *Strangulation of the:* The presence of this dangerous form of hernia is shown by a painful incompressible swelling, desire to go to stool with an inability to pass anything except what may have been in the bowel beneath the seat of the rupture previous to the occurrence of the strangulation. Efforts must be made to push the tumours back into the abdomen. A copious injection of tepid water has been known to facilitate this. If this fail one end of a table should be raised so as to form a steep inclined plane. The patient should then be held on this with his head much below the level of his feet. Pressure should be exerted on the swelling while he is in this position. A gurgling sound will herald the return of the protrusion to its proper place. A compress of *Blue* El. should be placed over the seat of hernia and a truss applied over this. The patient should take *Scrof.* alt. *Canc 5.* Compress of *Lord.* Apply *Red* alt. *Yellow* El. to 18 and 5. (4.) *Tubercle of the* (Scrofulous disease of the intestines): The presence of this disease is indicated by frequent or persistent intestinal catarrh and wasting. For treatment see Mesenteritis.

Brain, Abscess in the: This is the usual termination of local Cerebritis (inflammation of the brain substance) when this is caused by bone disease, injury, or pyæmia. Usually it is single, but there are sometimes several small abscesses. For treatment see Cerebritis. (1.) *Concussion of:* Probably *Feb. 1*, second dil., alt. *Scrof. 1*, second dil. Compress of *White* or *Blue* El. *Canc. 5* lotion. (2.) *Effusion*: Following malignant fever. *Scrof.* alt. *Canc. 5* alt. *Ang.* dil. Baths *Scrof.* alt. *Canc. 5.* Compresses *Scrof. 1* alt. *Canc. 5*, and *Red* El. alt. *Blue* El. to head. (3.) *Fag:* *Scrof. 1* third dil. Baths of *Scrof.* alt. *Canc. 5* alt. *White* or *Green* El. Unctions *Scrof.* or *Canc. 5.* Compresses *Scrof.* alt. *Canc. 5.* (4.) *Inflammation of:* See Cerebritis. (5.) *Softening of the:* Patients for some time suffer from depression of spirits, loss of memory, dullness of expression. This is often followed by Paralysis or semi-Paralysis. *Canc.*, second dil. alt. *Ang.* third dil. 1 glob. *Canc. 5* hourly. *Scrof.* at meals. *Blue* or *Green* El. to the six points and crown of the head. Baths of *Canc. 5* alt. *Ang. 2* alt. *Scrof.* or of *White*, *Red* or *Blue* El. Ointments, *Canc. 5*, *Ang. 3*, *Scrof. 5* to head, and *Feb. 2* to 24. Compresses,

changes from clear frothy mucus to a more opaque, viscid and sometimes even purulent substance. There is cough, the breathing is interfered with, and there is more or less feverishness. When the inflammation extends into the minute capillary tubes the breathing is very greatly disturbed; cough is exceedingly frequent and violent; expectoration is difficult; the countenance becomes pale and the expression anxious, and the temperature rises considerably, sometimes to 103° or more. Treatment: 1. *Acute Bronchitis:* Attack the fever *Feb. 1* second dil. and *Feb. 2* to 24. Afterwards give *Pet. 1* or *4*, litre dil. taking this in alternation with *Feb. 1* second dil. while any feverishness remains. Care must be taken to change the dilution of *Pet. 1* to the second or even third if any aggravation is caused. If the sputum is streaked with blood give a quarter glass of *Ang. 1* or *Ang. 3* in teaspoonfuls of the second dil. during the day. Compresses of *Red* or *Blue* El. on the chest are useful. When the inflammation subsides take *Pet. 1*, litre dil. alt. *Scrof. 1*, litre dil. and afterwards *Scrof. 1* first dil. only. 2. *Capillary Bronchitis:* Same treatment, with *Ang. 1* third dil. *Blue* El. on chest. 3. *Chronic Bronchitis:* Same treatment as the acute form. 4. *Chronic Bronchitis with Asthma:* Alternate *Pet. 3* second dil. and *Scrof. 1* second dil. with the remedies suggested above.

Bruises: Apply small compresses of *Blue* or *White* El.

Bubo: An inflammatory tumour situated in the groin, armpit, neck or anus. Treatment—1. *For the Simple Form: Scrof.* second dil.; compresses, *Scrof.* alt. *Lin.*; baths, *Lin.* 2. *For the Syphilitic form: Ven.* alt. *Canc. 5* dil.; baths of *Ven.* alt. *Lin.*

Bulimy: Abnormal hunger, producing faintness if the craving for food is not satisfied. Hysterical and pregnant females are its chief victims. *Scrof.* dil.; 3 globs. *Scrof. 1* dry three times a day. *Red* El. to 6. Baths of *Lin.*

Bunion: An enlarged bursa, generally on the great toe, usually caused by the foolish habit of wearing narrow-toed boots. Treatment: Use properly made boots. Take *Scrof. 1*, first dil., and apply ointment of *Canc. 5* or *Scof. 1.*

Burns or Scalds: Compresses of *Red* or *White* El. covered by compress of *Scrof. 3*, and take *Scrof. 1* first dil. *Red* El. however, should not be used when the skin is broken. *Canc. 5* oil is also very serviceable. The injured part should be covered so as to exclude the air. Dressings should be seldom changed in severe cases.

Buzzing in Ears. See Ears.

Calculus (Stone): A hard concretion lodged in some duct or passage. The term is commonly applied either to biliary calculi (gall stones) which are formed in the gall-bladder or biliary-ducts, or to urinary calculi, which are deposited in the kidneys or bladder. 1. *Biliary Calculi* are usually composed of crystalized bile. Occasionally they are very numerous; sometimes several are united in a compact mass. They often set up irritation or inflammation. If they lodge in the liver they sometimes produce abscesses. Other evil results may follow from their presence, such as obstruction of the bile-duct or intestines, inflammation or ulceration of the bowels, &c. They are expelled with the stools. As a rule their passage along the ducts to the intestines produces excruciating colicky pains (hepatic colic) of a griping burning nature, which shoot over the abdomen and up the back. There are also faintness, exhaustion, and sometimes vomiting or hiccough. Treatment: *Scrof. 2* alt. *Feb. 1* second dil. Every morning take 10 globs. *Feb. 1* dry on the tongue, and apply *Feb. 2* ointment to 24 night and morning. Baths of *Scrof. 5* alt. *Feb. 2* are also decidedly beneficial, as are compresses of *Feb. 2* 10 globs., alt. *Canc. 2* 10 globs. Some Matteists recommend commencing the treatment with *Scrof. 1* in dil. and afterwards passing on to *Scrof. 2*. After the calculus has disappeared use *Scrof. 1* first dil. to prevent the formation of new ones. 2. *Urinary Calculi:* These are derived from a deposit from the urine. There are several varieties, including those formed of uric acid, urates, oxalate of lime, &c. The commonest are those formed of uric acid. These are believed to owe their origin primarily to inactivity of the liver, and the resultant extra strain put upon the kidneys. The uric acid or lithic deposit first reveals itself in the form of particles in the urine resembling red sand or cayenne pepper. If there is much of this it is termed red gravel. In time the deposit increases, and a stone is formed. The urates when first noticed resemble brick dust. Young children are the chief victims of this form of calculus. The presence of stone leads to increased micturation, pains at the end of the urethra during and after the passage of water, occasional stoppage in the flow of water, appearance in the urine of muco-pus, and occasionally of blood, and a and deepening of the colour of the urine. The passage of stone from the kidney to the bladder gives rise to excruciating pain, and sometimes to laceration of the membrane of the urethra. Treatment: First or litre dil. *Scrof. 1* or *Scrof. 5* (in some cases) or of *Scrof. 1* alt. *Ang. 3* litre or second dil. Take 3 to 5 globs. *Scrof. 1* or *Scrof. 5* at meals. Apply *White* El. compresses to 20, 22, 25, and *Red* and *Yellow* El. to 5, 6, 12, 17, 18 and the kidney region. Ointment of *Feb. 2* to 24, and *Canc. 5* to the abdomen, kidney region, 20 and 25. Compresses of *Scrof. 1* to the kidney region, and baths of *Scrof. 5* alt. *Canc. 5* are also of service. The Mattei remedies will dissolve the stone. Sufferers from the disease should use little animal food or wine.

CANCER: A collection of cells ot a malignant character, having a tendency to infect the whole system of the patient in whom it occurs. The cancer first assumes the form of a small hard gland which is not sensitive to the touch, remains stationary for a time, and if it is situated near the surface of the body is often readily moveable. After a while it gradually increases in volume, adheres to the overlying skin and becomes fixed. By degrees it infiltrates the surrounding textures and glands and gives rise to lancinating pains. The skin over it becomes discoloured, and the whole system gradually becomes affected. A straw-coloured tint spreads over the body. Weight decreases. In many cases the edges of the tumour next become hard and ragged, its interior becomes dark, and a fœtid discharge flows from it, which at first is thick, but gradually grows thinner as the disease progresses. In some instances, however, no ulceration occurs, and in a great many cases no softening takes place. There are numerous varieties of Cancer, of which the chief are Scirrhus, or hard cancer, sometimes called stony cancer, which appears most frequently in the breast, stomach and womb; Encephaloid or soft cancer; Epithelioma, which chiefly affects the lips, tongue, and male genital organs; Hæmatoid, or bleeding cancer, and Melanotic or black cancer, which is almost always multiple in its character. The commonest seats of cancer are the female breast, the uterus, the lip, the intestines, the stomach, and the tonsils. The brain, liver, gullet, lymphatic glands, genital organs, kidneys, &c., are also occasional seats of this terrible disease. The presence of a cancer in an external part of the body may be evident to the eye and hand. In many instances, however, it is extremely difficult to determine whether a visible or tangible tumour is or is not of a malignant type. Many persons believe themselves to be suffering from cancer who are only affected by cysts, fatty or fibrous tumours, hypertrophy of the glands, &c. Hence the importance of submitting every doubtful case to the scrutiny of a competent practitioner. In the case of internal tumours the diagnosis is still more difficult. It may, however, be noted that Cancer in the *Stomach* leads to neuralgic pains in the stomach and back, eructations and the vomiting of a coffee-like substance, and that externally the tumour becomes perceptible to the touch. Cancer in the *Liver* leads to an increase of the size of this organ, dyspepsia, jaundice, dropsy, and dull lancinating pains in the right side of the hypochondriac region, which shoot up to the shoulder and then down the right arm. Afterwards there is diarrhœa, accompanied by the straw-coloured tint of the body to which we have already referred. Cancer in the *Kidney* produces severe pains in the lumbar region, which generally shoot towards the thigh, and bleeding from the kidneys. Cancer in the *Uterus* produces hæmorrhage, and shooting pains, and is accompanied by a discharge possessing a peculiarly disagreeable odour. Those who believe themselves to be in danger of cancer should use the following :—

1. PREVENTIVE TREATMENT. — Twice daily take from 2 to 5 globs. *Scrof. Giap.* During five weeks in autumn and spring take *Canc. 1* first dil., three-quarters of a tumblerful during each day, in frequent teaspoonfuls, *i.e.*, about every half hour. Towards the critical age women should alternate *Ang. 1* with *Canc. 1.* This will prevent uterine congestions.

Those who actually suffer from cancer or from non-malignant tumours should use the following :—

2. CURATIVE TREATMENT.—N.B.: The dilutions and compresses are essential. The other parts of the treatment will accelerate the cure.

A.—INTERNAL TREATMENT.

At first.—Take *Ang. 3* or *Ang. 1* second dil. during the morning, half a tumblerful in teaspoonfuls at short intervals. If this excites the heart use the third dil., and if this is too stimulating to the circulatory system take only six or eight teaspoonfuls per diem.

In the afternoon women should take *Canc. 1* second dil., or the third dil. if the second increases the cancer pains. In uterine cancers the third dil. is generally the best. After a few days the stronger dilutions may be tried. Men may take the litre dil. at first, and afterwards the first dil. In any case, nearly half a tumblerful of the proper dilution should be taken in frequent teaspoonfuls from 2 to 10 p.m. The strength of dilution that can be borne should be ascertained before the use of dry globules is added to the treatment. Otherwise the dilutions may erroneously be supposed to be at fault. Every hour take 1 dry glob. of *Canc. 1*, and 5 globs. *Canc. 1* at one or more meals. Or men may take from 5 to 10 globs. and women from 3 to 5 globs. of *Canc. 4* dry on the tongue night and morning.

If the patient suffer from indigestion he should take 3 to 5 globs. of *Scrof. 5* dry on tongue each morning and 2 to 3 after each meal; or he may take 5 globs. *Scrof. Giap.* in the beverage at meals once or twice a day. If there is any feverishness let him take a teaspoonful of *Feb. 1* second dil. every half-hour till it disappears. As the liver is generally more or less deranged 2 globs. *Feb. 1* may be given after meals, or 2 globs. at bedtime.

Subsequently.—Gradually increase the doses if this can be borne. If, however, *Canc. 1* and *Ang. 1* or *3* have produced insufficient results, *Canc. 5* first dil. alt. *Ang. 2* litre or second dil., with 1 glob. *Canc. 2* every hour, and 10 globs. *Canc. 1* in the beverages at meals twice a day may be tried. Or progress may be hastened by giving 2 globs. *Canc. 4* before each meal, and giving *Ang. 2* alt. *Canc. 5* in dil.

Be careful to *stir or shake up* the dilutions before using.

If, after signs of improvement have been seen, the

curative process should suddenly cease the patient should take 10 to 20 globs. *Canc. 5* dry on the tongue in a single dose once daily for a week. The effects of this strong dose should be carefully marked. It should not be repeated if evil ensues. Should this fail a few doses of *Verm.* or of *Ven.* should be given, as the failure may arise either from the presence of worms or from an inherited or acquired syphilitic taint.

B.—EXTERNAL TREATMENT.

I.—COMPRESSES.

(i.) Closed Tumours.— Place on the tumour a large compress which has been soaked in water medicated with 15 to 25 globs. of *Canc. 1*, or with 15 to 20 globs. of *Canc. 5* to every 6 ounces of water, *i.e.*, about three-quarters of a tumblerful. Cover this with some water-proof material. Bind the whole together with a flannel bandage. If the use of water-proof material causes irritation use the flannel only. After ascertaining what strength of *Canc.* lotion the patient can bear, a smaller compress, moistened with *Red* El. or *Red* El. and water (10 drops to a tablespoonful) may be placed on the tumour beneath the larger compress.

(ii.) Ulcerated Tumours.—Place on the tumour a small linen rag which has been soaked in *Green* El. and water, in the proportion of 10 drops of *Green* El. to each tablespoonful of water. Cover this, as in the previous case, with a large compress moistened with water medicated with *Canc. 5.* Waterproof material should not be used in these cases.

2.—BATHS.

After a few days' internal treatment the patient may in most cases, advantageously take warm baths medicated with *Ang. 3* alt. *Canc. 5*, 50 to 100 globs. being dissolved in half a pint of water, which is then poured into the bath. If the patient is highly nervous, baths of *Feb. 2* will calm him.

The patient should remain in the bath from 5 to 20 minutes. In uterine cases, sitz-baths are useful, 30 globs. to the bath.

Care should be taken to avoid chills after baths.

The effect of the dilutions upon the functions should be observed before taking the baths.

If the bath cannot be borne sponge the spine well over with a lotion made by dissolving 10 globs. *Canc. 5* or *Canc. 6* in a quarter of a pint of brandy. Or a liniment may be made by dissolving in a one ounce bottle 10 to 15 globs. of *Scrof. 5* in 1 drachm of *White* El. and 3 drachms of glycerine, and filling up with water. Gently rub this over the spine with the hand.

3.— INJECTIONS.

In uterine tumours, injections of tepid water, medicated with *Canc. 2* or *Canc. 5* (10 globs. to the half-pint) or *Ang. 2* are sometimes useful. When suitable, *Green* or *Blue* El. may be added.

4.—GARGLES AND INHALATIONS.

Gargles or sprays of *Canc. 1*, *Ang. 1*, *White* El. or *Green* El. are useful in mouth and throat cases, and inhalations of the same remedies in nose cases.

It must be borne in mind that *if pain increases under treatment the dose must be diminished*, and that the more sensitive the patient is, either naturally or in consequence of the disease, the weaker should be the doses. As the doses are weakened their frequency should generally be increased.

In some cases it has been found better to put the *Canc. 5* compress around rather than over the smaller compress.

The wound may be bathed with a lotion made by dissolving 10 globs. *Canc. 1* or *Scrof. 1* in three ounces of tepid water.

(iii.) Bleeding Tumours.—Soak the smaller rag in *Blue* El. instead of in *Red* or *Green*, as in the previous cases, and cover it as before with a *Canc. 5* compress.

In cases of hæmorrhage the lint with which the wound has been dressed should be wetted with a lotion made by dissolving 10 globs. of *Ang. 2* in half a tumblerful of tepid water. The wound should then be well sponged with the lotion, and, if necessary, plugs of scraped lint saturated with it should be introduced into the cavities from which the blood spurts out. After this, the wound should be bathed with a similar lotion of *Canc.* Compresses dipped in the *Ang. 2* lotion and others in the *Canc.* lotion, should be spread alternately over the wound. If there is no bleeding use *Canc.* alone.

5.—ELECTRICITIES.

Violent pains will disappear on applying *Green* El. to the tumour. This may also be taken internally, a drop being put into a quart of water and teaspoonful doses taken occasionally.

Lymphatic patients may tone up their nervous system by applying *Red* El. by means of a small sponge inserted into the neck of the bottle, to the sympathetic, solar plexus, occiput, pit of the stomach, and to all the nerves corresponding with the tumour. The application to each point should last from 5 to 10 seconds. As soon as the points are dry, *Yellow* El. should be applied to them. 5 drops of *White* or *Blue* El. may be poured on the crown of the head every morning.

Sanguine patients should use *Blue* El. instead of *Red* and *Yellow*.

6.—OINTMENTS.

(i.) Once to three times a day, in cases of *closed tumours*, or of infiltrated glands in their neighbourhood, *Canc. 5* ointment may be gently applied to them. *Ointment, however, should never be applied to an open wound.*

(ii.) Two or three times a day, *Ang. 3* ointment may be gently applied to the heart. This will improve the circulation —a matter of great importance to a victim of cancer.

(iii.) Two or three times a day, *Feb. 2* ointment should be well rubbed over the hypochondria (marked 24 in diagram) for 3 or 4 minutes at a time. This will tone up the liver and spleen.

When the treatment is successful the sore loses its fœtor, pain diminishes and then dies away, the gland becomes smaller, its discolouration diminishes, it softens and becomes less adherent. By degrees it becomes slightly sensitive. The suppuration thickens and assumes a yellowish tint. And, after a time, fragments of the diseased substance become detached or the whole tumour falls off in a mass.

When an external cancerous wound begins to cicatrize

the healing process may be hastened by the application of compresses of *Scrof. 1* or *6*, and injections into the wound of *Scrof. 6* lotion. When the whole tumour has been detached *Canc. 2* may be substituted for *Canc. 1* until the cicatrization is complete, and then *Scrof. 1* must be regularly taken for several weeks.

Count Mattei maintains that while the suppuration is abundant and thick there is hope of recovery.

Cases which are beyond hope of cure may be relieved both of the distressing pain and of the disagreeable fœtor by the application of compresses of *Green* El. and the use of the treatment prescribed above.

Cancrum Oris (Canker of mouth): Gangrenous or sloughing ulcer which chiefly affects ill-fed or tuberculous children. Morning and evening 2 globs. of *Canc. 1* or of *Ven.* dry on the tongue. During the morning *Ang. 3* second dil.; during the afternoon, *Canc. 1* second dil. Compresses of *Green* El. and *Scrof. 5* or *Lin.* to the ulcers. Baths of *Canc. 5*.

Carbuncle: A fiery inflammation causing burning pain. The tumour itself is hard but tender, it is of a circular flat shape, of a dusky red colour, and discharges from several openings. Take *Canc. 1* or *4* in dil., alt. *Ang. 1.* second dil.; 5 globs. *Lin.* dry on the tongue night and morning. Compresses of *Canc. 1* or *5* and *Green* El. 2 drops of *Blue* El. on sugar once a day. Occasional compresses of *Scrof. 1* and *Ang. 2* have been found useful. *Red* and *Yellow* El. may be applied alternately to the corresponding nerves. After the tumour has subsided *Ang. 2* or *3* should be used daily for some time.

In simple *Anthrax* the fever should be subdued by

Feb. 1 second dil. and the treatment suggested above carried out in all respects.

Carditis; A rare disease consisting in inflammation of the muscular walls of the heart. *Ang. 3* second or third dil. alt. *Canc. 1* third dil. 3 globs. *Scrof. 2* at meals. Warm compresses of *Ang. 3* (2 globs. to a tablespoonful of water) may be applied to the heart, and *Feb. 2* ointment to 24.

Cardialgia: Better known as Heartburn, which see.

Caries: Ulceration of bones, the particles of bone being absorbed or being carried away in a purulent discharge. *Canc. 4* first or intermediate dil., *Scrof. 1* and *5* at meals. Compresses of *Green* El. alt. *Canc. 5* or *Canc. 4*.

Caries of Nasal Bone. Same treatment as above with inhalations of *Canc. 1*, *4* or *5*, and compresses of *Canc. 5* to the diseased parts.

Caries of the Teeth: Alt. *Scrof. 1* and *Canc. 4* in litre dil. Gargles of *Canc. 5* alt. *Ang. 3*. *Canc. 5* ointment to jaws.

Catalepsy: a statue-like fixedness of the body with impaired sensation, frequently accompanied by insensibility. *Red* El. to 11 and 18 usually suffices. Should this be insufficient apply *Canc. 5* ointment to 11, and give *Canc. 1* second dil. Baths of *White* El. or *Blue* El. according to the temperament of patient.

Cataract: an opaque condition of the lens of the eye, of the lens and capsule of the lens, or of the latter only. *Scrof. 1*, second or third dil. alt. *Ang. 1* second or third dil. if there is any congestion of the head or eyes. After a month, if there is no improvement, take *Canc. 1* or *5*, third dil. Apply *Canc. 5* ointment alt. *Scrof. 5* ointment alt. *Ang. 3* ointment to the whole head. *Feb. 2* ointment or *Canc. 5* ointment to 24. Baths of *Canc. 5* alt. *Scrof. 5* alt. *Ang. 3.* *Red* El. to 11, 2, 3, *Red* El. alt. *Yellow* to 11, 18, 2, 3, 23, and 1. When the opacity decreases the eye should be shielded from the light.

Catarrh, acute: a cold which generally attacks the nostrils first and may afterwards pass to the chest. At the outset take 1 glob. *Scrof. 1* dry on the tongue each quarter of an hour, for two or three hours in succession, or take in one dose 3 globs. in 3 oz. of water. Should it fail or should the use of it have been begun too late take *Pet. 3* in the litre dil. or dry alt. with *Scrof. Giap.* first dil. or *Scrof. 1* or, if there is any fever, with *Feb. 1,* first or lit. dil. Apply *Pet. 3* ointment and *Red* El. to the root of the nose, also *Feb. 2* ointment to 24. It is necessary to watch the effects of *Pet.*, as if taken too often it sometimes causes sneezing. It should then be alt. with *Canc. 1.* Afterwards *Scrof. 1* or *Scrof. 2* may be taken dry and *Scrof. 5* ointment applied to root of nose, throat, chest ,&c.

Catarrh of Bladder. See Cystitis.
" *Bronchial.* See Bronchitis.
" *Gastric.* See Gastritis.
" *Intestinal.* See Enteritis.
" *Laryngeal.* See Laryngitis.
" *Pharyngeal.* See Pharyngitis.
" *Pulmonary.* See Pneumonia.
" *Uterine.* See Womb.

Chilblain : An inflammation of the skin of the fingers or toes, caused by exposure to damp or cold. The tendency to chillblains may be counteracted by *Ang. 2* second dil. When chillblains appear, take *Scrof. 1* first dil., and apply *Canc. 5*, *Scrof.* or *Ang. 2* ointment. Compresses of *Red*, *Blue* or *White* El., or of *Canc. 5* or *Scrof. 1* may also be used. Baths of *Canc. 5*, *Scrof. 1* or *Lin.*

Cephalagia : See Headache.

Cephalematoma, may be dispersed by compresses of *Ang. 1.* or, if suppurating, of *Ang. 2* alt. *Canc. 5.*

Chancre : A Syphilitic sore. For treatment see Syphilis.

Change of Life : To prevent the congestions, &c., which usually trouble ladies at this time take *Scrof. 2* second dil. alt. *Ang. 3* litre or second dil. 2 globs. *Lin.* every morning after breakfast. 1 glob. *Canc. 1* every 2 hours. *Verm.* is often needed as an intercurrent remedy, especially by women with wheezy stomach cough. Baths of *Canc. 5* (100 globs.) Injections of *Ang.* (20 globs. to half-pint.) *Lin.* ointment for back, from waist down, and *Canc. 5* ointment for abdomen.

Chapped Hands : Often caused by partial drying of hands or use of strong soaps. Internally *Scrof. 1* first dil. or *Canc. 1* litre dil., with *Canc. 5* compresses. The following is a useful lotion. In a 1 oz. bottle dissolve 20 globs. of *Scrof. 5* in 1 drachm *White* El. and 1 drachm of glycerine. Shake well up and fill with boiled water. Use after washing and always shake before applying.

Chapped Nipples : To prevent, sponge the bosoms daily for six weeks before accouchement with cold lotion of *Scrof. 1*, or in a little water take 3 globs. *Scrof. 1* night and morning.

Cheek (Swollen) : *Scrof. 1* second dil., 5 globs. *Scrof. Giap.* at meals. *Red* El. or *Red* alt. *Yellow* El. to 3, 18 and under ear.

Chicken-pox: An acute eruption resembling small-pox. There are small pointed vesicles which become filled with watery fluid, dry up about the third day and form crusts or scabs. *Scrof. 1* first dil. alt. *Feb.* second dil. Compress of *Feb. 2* to 24, or ointment of *Feb. 2* to 24.

Chill: When first felt take 10 globs. *Scrof. 1* or *Scrof. Giap.* (or *5* if the patient is of a billious temperament), and repeat the dose a few minutes afterward. Should this fail to produce a glow apply *Red, White* or *Blue* El. to the centre of the cranium and base of nose. Should feverishness ensue take *Feb. 1* in the litre dil. Apply compresses of *White* El. or *Feb. 2* to 24. After the fever has passed away take *Scrof. 1* third dil.; apply *Red* and *Yellow* El. to 18 and 17, and take a bath of *Canc. 5.*

Chiragia (Gout in the hand): See Gout.

Chlorosis: A peculiar form of anæmia, accompanied by deficiency of blood and of red corpuscles. There is a peculiar greenish-yellow hue on the patient's face. Temperature is diminished. The action of the heart is easily disturbed, menstruation is imperfect, and the whole body is debilitated. Sometimes there is puffiness of the eyes and swelling of the ankles. Often there is hysterical pain, especially in the left side. Noises in the ear, headache, and costiveness are frequently complained of. There is generally great distaste, if not absolute disgust, for food. Treatment: Same as in Anæmia.

Cholera, Asiatic: a violent acute disease, which commences by vomiting, diarrhœa, resembling rice-water, and a feeling of great prostration at the pit of the stomach. There are great restlessness and thirst, cramps, a rapid pulse, a feeling of intense heat but an actual lowness of temperature. As the patient collapses the temperature rises above normal.

Preventive treatment: Take 5 globs. of *Scrof. Giap.* dry on the tongue once or twice a day. Avoid much fruit and carefully follow the laws of health.

Curative treatment: Take 20 globs. of *Scrof. Giap.* or *Scrof. 1* dry on the tongue, and 1 glob. of *Scrof. Giap.* or *Scrof.* every five minutes, or give *Scrof. Giap.* first dil. every five minutes. Apply *Red* or *White* El. to 6, 18, 17, and warm compresses of *Canc. 5* on abdomen. If the disease is obstinate, try baths of *Canc. 5*, *Ang. 3* or *White* El. During convalesence give *Scrof. Giap.* first dil. Apply compress of *Feb. 2* to 24. Baths of *Canc. 5* alt. *Scrof. 1*. Apply *Red* alt. *Yellow* El. to 6, 18, 17.

Infantile: Give *Canc. 6* in the second dil. alt. with *Scrof. Giap.* in the first or lit. dil., in half-teaspoonful doses. The child should only be allowed barley or rice water, into which the white of an egg may have been introduced.

Cholerine: A violent form of diarrhœa, resembling Cholera in many respects, which prevails during epidemics of Cholera. At the outset take 20 globs. of *Scrof. 1* or *Scrof. Giap.* and afterwards small doses of *Scrof. 1* in the first dil.

Chorea: A disturbance of the nervous system, accompanied by what has been well designated as insanity of the muscles. The patient loses control over the motor apparatus. His muscular movements are excessive, but weak and wanting in precision. Chorea arises from rheumatism, fright, worms, teething, or even, as some suppose, from watching the movements of those who are subject to it. *Scrof.* second dil. alt. *Verm.* or *Ang.* second dil. if worms on the one hand or defective circulation on the other are supposed to give rise to it. Only one to six teaspoonfuls of each remedy should be taken during the day. *Canc.* 5 may be tried in obstinate cases. Other useful remedies include *Lin.*, *Scrof.* 2 in second or third dil.; *Red* alt. *Yellow* El. to 5, 18, 17; *Scrof.* 5 compresses to the muscles most affected; ointment of *Canc.* 5 to the head and *Ang.* 3 to the heart; and baths of *Canc.* 5, *Scrof.* 1 or 5 or *Lin.*

Cirrhosis: See Liver.

Cold: See Chills and Catarrh.

Colic: Spasmodic contraction of the muscular coat of the large intestine, giving rise to paroxysms of griping pain, which lead the patient to writhe and roll and often to double himself up. His extremities become cold, he becomes depressed and agitated. There is no fever. The disease may be distinguished from hernia by there being no tumour, and from enteritis by there being no extreme tenderness, but, on the contrary, relief, on the application of pressure. 1 glob. *Scrof.* 1 dry every five minutes: *Scrof.* 1 alt. *Canc.* 5 both in first dil; warm compresses of *Canc.* 5 to abdomen; *Red* or *White* El. to 6; warm baths of *Canc.* 5, or *Canc.* 5 ointment to 6 and abdomen may be tried.

Colic, Hepatic: This is distinguished from other forms by beginning in the right hypochondrium, and shooting round to the back and over the right shoulder. For treatment see Gall stones.

Colic, Nephritic : Due to the passage of a calculus from the kidney to the bladder. Characterised by sudden shooting agonising pains, which proceed from the renal region towards the bladder and thence outwards, and producing clammy sweats and faintness. For treatment see Calculus (Renal.)

Colic, Menstrual : See Menstruation, Painful.

Coma : Suspension of consciousness, resulting from narcotic poisoning, congestion of the brain, or its membranes, etc. In its most fatal forms the breathing is slow and noisy, the eye is insensible to light. The patient should be placed with his head a little raised, the garments about his neck should be loosened, and, if there is a suspicion of poisoning, the stomach-pump should be used. If it arises from congestion of the brain, treat like apoplexy. If from meningitis, like that disease.

Congestion of the Brain : Caused by interference with the escape of blood out of the brain by the excessive action of the heart, or by excess of blood in the whole system. There is dull headache at the crown and back of the head, a confusion of thought, and a tendency to vertigo. The patient grows drowsy, he hears various noises in his head, sees specks before his eyes, and feels pain in the limbs. Very often there are muscular twitchings. *Ang.* second dil. alt., in very grave cases, with *Canc. 1* in the second or third dil. *Blue* El. should be applied to the chief nerve centres in the head. If the congestion is serious, treat as in apoplexy.

Congestion of Liver : Resulting from exposure to extreme heat or cold, wrong diet, injury, etc., accompanied by a dull heavy pain in the neighbourhood of the liver, and a sharp pain in the right shoulder. The tongue is foul and the appetite impaired. There is often slight jaundice. At the outset take 10 globs. *Feb. 1* dry on the tongue, afterwards *Feb. 1* in second dil. Ointment of *Feb. 2.* alt. *Canc. 5* to 24. Application of *Red* alt. *Yellow* El. to 5, 18, 17, 24. Baths of *Feb. 2*, *Canc. 5*, *Ang. 3* are also useful.

Congestion of the Lungs: This may result from heart disease, etc. It produces a sense of tightness across the chest. *Pet. 1* second dil. alt *Ang. 1* third dil., with compress of *Ang. 2* to the heart and left side of the lungs. If the congestion should be followed by yellowish-green expectoration alt. *Pet. 2* or *3* second dil. with *Canc. 1* or *5* in the second dil., and *Ang. 1* in the third dil.

Constipation: Sluggish action of the intestines, resulting from defective secretion of the juices of the mucous membrane of the bowels, or from feeble contraction of the muscular fibres. Sometimes it is caused by congestion of the portal system, by improper diet, by sedentary habits, or by the use of aperients. Purgatives should be avoided. Litre or second dil. of *Scrof. 1* or of *Scrof. 5* in bilious temperaments, or *Canc. 5*, third dil. with 5 to 10 dry globs. of *Scrof. 1* every morning. Sanguine patients require 5 to 10 globs. *Ang. 3* every morning dry or in beverage at breakfast, with *Ang. 3* dil. When the liver is affected take *Feb. 1*, second dil. alt. *Canc. 1*, second or third dil., and apply *Feb. 2* ointment to 24. In many cases it is advantageous to take 3 globs. of *Verm.* in a tumblerful of water every morning for a fortnight. It should be drunk in 1 to 4 draughts. In most cases compresses or ointments of *Canc. 5* to the abdomen, or the pouring of *Canc. 5* lotion over the abdomen will be found extremely useful. Patients who suffer from costiveness should remember that those who are habitually costive are usually longer lived than those who habitually suffer from diarrhœa. They should take brown bread, oatmeal porridge, oleaginous articles, cocoa, and ripe fruit, especially at breakfast. A couple of bananas may with great advantage be eaten before breakfast. Patients should form the habit of going to stool at a regular hour every day, and should use tepid enemata of *Lin.*, *Canc. 5*, *Feb. 2*, or *Ang. 1* dissolved in a teaspoonful each of glycerine and water, which may be introduced by means of the glycerine syringe.

Consumption : a deposition of albuminous matter or tubercles in various parts of the body, especially in the lungs and mesenteric glands, associated with a morbid state of the digestive organs. The chief symptoms are dry cough, with subsequent expectoration of a little clear frothy fluid and afterwards of yellow or greyish matter, tightness across and pains in the chest, acceleration of the pulse, and nocturnal perspirations. At a later stage the expectoration becomes greenish-yellow and is occasionally tinged with blood, a hectic flush appears, the cough increases, breathing becomes more difficult, the chest flattens, the tubercles form ulcers which destroy the neighbouring tissues, portions of the diseased lung are expectorated, obstinate diarrhœa, and hectic fever set in and the patient becomes emaciated and dies. During first stage *Scrof. 2* second dil. alt. *Pet. 2* second dil., with *Pet. 3* ointment on chest. At meals take globs. of *Scrof. 1* or *Scrof. Giap.* As soon as the expectoration becomes streaked, substitute *Ang. 2* second dil. for *Scrof. 2*. When the night sweats begin, alternate *Canc. 1* or *4* second dil. with the other remedies, and apply *Canc. 5* or *Lin.* ointment on chest, *Ang. 2* or *3* to the heart, and *Feb. 2* to 24. Should this not subdue the fever, give a few teaspoonfuls of *Feb. 1*, in the third dil., every evening. Apply *White* El. to 5, 18, 17. Should there be any laryngeal complications use gargles of *Pet. 3* alt. *Canc. 5*. Careful attention must be paid to diet, which should be nutritious and digestible. Albuminous food is specially required. The patient should breathe as deeply as possible, and should use inhalations of oxygen gas. If this cannot be done he must take deep inhalations of the purest atmospheric air to which he can have access.

Contraction of Hand: Take *Scrof. 1* in litre dil. Apply *Red*, *Yellow*, or *Green* El. to nerves of hand. Compresses and ointments of *Canc. 5*, *Scrof. 1* or *White* El.

Contraction of Nerves: *Scrof. 1*, litre dil. *Red* alt. *Yellow* El. to 5, 18, 17. Baths of *Lin. Canc. 5*, *White* El.

Convalescence: As a tonic during convalescence, take first dil. of *Scrof. 1* or *Scrof. 5*. Take 2 globs. *Scrof. 1* three times a day, and 3 to 5 drops *White* El. in a wineglassful of water between meals. Apply *Red* alt. *Yellow* El. to the chief nerve centres.

Convulsions: Convulsive movements of various kinds occasioned by over-work, various organic diseases of the brain, meningeal effusion of blood, irritation from worms, etc. They chiefly attack young children and women, and are sometimes associated with measles, meningitis, and other acute diseases. The muscular movements are sudden, irregular and involuntary. In the treatment of the disease the cause must always be considered In the majority of cases, *Scrof.* in the second dil. or *Scrof. 2* in the second or third dil. may be given internally, six or eight spoonfuls being administered during the day. If disorders of the circulation are supposed to cause them baths of *Ang. 3* in the third dil. may be prescribed. When worms originate the disease *Ver. 1* in the third dil. must be taken; 1 drop of *Yellow* El. in a teaspoonful of water each morning. In many cases *Yellow* El. may be applied to 5 and 6. When women are attacked *Canc. 1* should be alt. with *Ang. 3*, especially if there is any hysterical tendency.

Convulsive Movements: *Scrof. 1* second dil. Baths of *Canc. 5* alt. *White* El.

Cornea, Stains in: See Eyes.

Corns: A thickening of the epidermis, caused by undue pressure and friction, generally resulting from wearing ill-fitting boots. Compresses of *Scrof. 5*, *Canc. 5*, *Red* or *White* El. *Canc. 5*, or *Scrof. 5* ointment. *Scrof 1* internally in first dil.

Coryza: See Catarrh, Cold.

Cough: A series of forcible expirations caused by irritation of the surface of the air tubes or of the nerves by which they are supplied. This irritation may be reflex, as when it originates in the stomach, ear, &c. Sometimes cough is caused by a long uvula or enlarged tonsil. Coughs vary greatly in character. The hysterical cough is of a barking character. The cough of pleurisy is catching and painful. In the first stage of consumption the cough consists of a slight hacking. In asthma the cough is spasmodic and suffocating.

Dry Cough: *Pet. 1*; drops of *Blue* El.

A massive dose of 5 to 10 globs. *Pet.* will provoke expectoration.

In *Bronchial Cough Verm.* is sometimes useful. It is also valuable in Hooping Cough.

Catarrhal Cough (result of a chill): *Feb.* alt. *Pet. 3* alt. *Scrof. 1* (or *Ang. 1* if there are symptoms of congestion) 3 drops *White* El.; *White* El. to 6.

Chronic Cough (simple): *Pet. 1* or *3*. *Canc. 5* oint. Drops and gargles of *White* El.

Chronic Cough (with expectoration): *Pet. 3* or 4. The former is specially adapted to children, as it is the gentlest of the series of pectorals.

Phthisical Cough: *Pet. 2*, second dil. alt. *Canc. 4*, second dil.; *Scrof. 2* at meals; *Canc. 5* ointment to chest; (See Consumption.)

Stomach Cough: *Scrof. 1*. *Red* El. to 6.

Whooping Cough: (See Hooping Cough.)

Worm Cough (Cough arising from the irritation caused by worms): *Verm.* third or litre dil. Drops of *Yellow* El. Gargles of *Verm. 2*. (See Worms.)

See Bronchitis, Croup, Diphtheria, Lungs, &c.

Coxalgia: See Hip Disease.

Cramp: A painful spasm chiefly affecting the calves of the legs, and often associated with irritation of the stomach or bowels. Those who are subject to it may take 10 globs. of *Scrof. 1* dry on the tongue at night, and apply lotions of *Scrof.* to the muscles which are most affected. *Red* and *Yellow* El. may be also applied to 5, 18, 17 in the case of cramp in the stomach, and to 11 in cramp in the head. For Writers' Cramp, ointment of *Canc. 5* or of *Scrof.* may be rubbed over the hand, and compresses of

Yellow or *Green* El. may be used. Cramp in the nerve of the heel may be relieved by *Red* El., and baths of *Canc. 5*. Cramp of the legs will be removed by ointment or compresses of *Canc. 5*, compresses of *White* El. or *Scrof. 5*., and baths of *Canc. 5* and *Scrof. 5*. In Menstrual Cramp, 10 globs of *Scrof.* may be given dry, and dil. of *Ang.* and *Scrof. 5* may afterwards be taken. 3 drops of *Blue* El. may be given on sugar. Compress of *Ang. 2* may be applied to 27 and the painful part, and *Scrof. 3* ointment may be gently applied down the groin.

Croup: What is usually known by this name is an inflammatory disease of the larynx or windpipe, or both, accompanied by the formation of a false membrane on the mucous membrane, and giving rise to stridulous breathing. It usually arises from exposure to chilly and damp airs and chiefly aflects infants. It is very dangerous. At first there are catarrh, feverishness and hoarseness. Breathing assumes a hissing character. A brassy cough is heard, and the patient is nearly suffocated. This form of croup is really diphtheria, and should be treated accordingly. (See Diphtheria.)

Fal·e Croup—Laryngismus Stridulus: Slight inflammation of the larynx and air passages. It may arise from any of the causes which can originate catarrh. It chiefly affects children and usually comes on at night. The child starts from sleep and coughs spasmodically with a cooing sound. During attack 5 globs. *Scrof. 1* every five minutes. *Domfin* first dil. a teaspoonful every five minutes or a dry glob. ever five minutes. *Red* El. compress to chin and neck. After the attack give *Scrof. 1* first or second dil.

Curvature of the Spine: See Spine.

Cutaneous Diseases: See under Eczema, Herpes, etc., also Skin Diseases.

Cuts: Compresses of *Ang. 3* or *Blue* El. may be used to stop the bleeding, and afterwards cicatrization may be promoted by means of *Scrof. 1* or *6.*

Cystitis—(Inflammation of the Bladder): In its acute form it may be caused by injuries, calculi, or by extension of inflammation from neighbouring parts. *Scrof. 6* second dil. or *Scrof 1* second dil. may be alt., with *Feb 2.* ointment to 24 so long as there is feverishness. A dry glob. of *Ang. 3* may be given each hour. Compress of *White* El. to 20, 22 and 25. *Red* alt. *Yellow* El. to 5, 11, 18 and 20. Tepid baths of *Ang. 3*, *Canc. 5* or *Scrof. 1.*

Cysts: A closed cavity containing fluid or soft matter. In some cases they are parasitic, but in the majority of cases they result from dilatation of previously existing closed cavities, from the obstruction of natural outlets of secreting organs, etc. Some forms of them easily become scirrhus or cancerous. Dil. of *Scrof. 1* alt. with *Canc. 1, 3* or *4.* When they are of long standing, ointment of *Canc. 5* and compresses of *Red* El.

Deafness: See Ear, Diseases of.

Debility: A state of weakness affecting the whole or a part of the body, commonly due to impaired nutrition. In most cases *Scrof. 1* in dil., with baths of *Canc. 5*, and application of the Electricities which best suit the temperament, to the six chief nerve centres in the case of general debility, or to the organs involved.

Delirium Tremens: A form of alcholism which begins with inability to take food, muscular tremor, etc., and is soon accompanied by tormenting visions, etc. *Scrof. 1* second dil. In some cases, *Ang.* with applications of *Red* El. to the right side of the great sympathetic, and *Yellow* El. to the left side, with *Red* and *Yellow* El. alt. to the gastric sympathetic, and centre of cranium.

Dentition, Difficult: *Scrof.* in second or third dil. If there is much irritation a compress of *Feb. 2* may be applied to 24.

Derryshire Neck : See Goitre.

Diabetes Insipidus : See Polyuria.

Diabetes Mellitus : An excessive flow of urine in which there is persistently present a considerable quantity of sugar. The patient at first notices that he has to pass water with increasing frequency, especially at night. This water is light in colour and of a peculiarly sweetish odour. Its specific gravity is high. The skin grows dry and harsh. A sçanty, sticky mucus covers the teeth, gums, and lips. Emaciation ensues. Appetite generally grows. Temperature becomes low, and sexual power is lost. Fever and diarrhœa supervene. Treatment : *Scrof. 1* or *Scrof. 6*, or, in obstinate cases, *Scrof. 6* alt. *Ang. 2* dil. alt. *Canc. 6* or *Canc. 1*. 2 globs. *Lin.* dry every morning. Applications of *Red*, *Yellow* or *Blue* El. to 5, 18, 17 and sides of spine, and ointment of *Feb. 2* to 24. *Lin.* and *Canc. 5* ointment to kidneys daily. Warm baths of *Canc. 5*, *Lin.*, *Scrof. 5* and *Ang. 3* or *Ang. 2*. Starchy foods and also substances containing cane or grape sugar should be avoided. Meat is regarded as the diabetic patient's staple article of diet. Green vegetables, nuts, watercress, lettuce, cocoa (from the nibs), gluten bread, and bran bread are permissible articles. Flannels should be worn next to the skin. Regular walking exercise should be taken.

Diarrhœa: Frequent and profuse evacuations resulting from direct irritation of the intestines, chill, nervous agitation, imperfectly digested food, foul emanations from decomposing matter, worms, &c. It accompanies several diseases such as Peritonitis, &c. At the outset take 5 dry globs. of *Scrof. Giap.* or *Scrof. 1.* Repeat the dose after each of four successive motions. Afterwards take *Scrof. Giap.* in first dil. alt. *Canc. 4* in first dil. Apply *Red* alt. *Yellow* El. to 5, 6, 17. Baths of *Canc. 5* or *Scrof. 5.* If there is blood in the stools give *Ang. 1* first or second dil. alt. *Scrof.* first or litre dil; 10 dry globs. of *Ang. 2* in a single dose, or 1 dry glob. per hour. Baths of *Ang. 3* alt. *Canc. 5.* In periodical diarrhœa alternate *Ang.* and *Scrof.*, replacing the latter by *Canc. 1* if this fails. Take 1 glob. *Scrof. Giap.* after each meal, and 2 globs. *Feb. 1* at night a day or two before the next attack is expected, In all cases of chronic diarrhœa *Scrof. 1* or *Scrof. Giap.* may be given in dry globules, and *Canc. 1* used both in dil. and in injections. Fruits, vegetables, hot food, animal broths, &c., should be avoided. Farinacea, white of egg, rice-water, milk and lime-water are allowable. In chronic cases a highly nutritious diet is important.

Diphtheria: A contagious and sometimes epidemic disease, characterised by exudation of a peculiar lymph, which, together with epithelial cells, forms a false membrane over the soft palate, uvula, tonsils, pharynx, &c. Patients who have had scarlatina are peculiarly liable to it. Children from 2 to 10 are the chief victims. The disease is a very dangerous one and must be treated with the utmost care. The invasion of the disease is insidious. Slight fever, huskiness, diarrhœa, and tickling cough are first noticed. Then follows an attack of stridulous breathing, sometimes a very sudden one, with great prostration of strength. Throat-examination reveals the false membrane. In many cases there are albuminuria or enlarged glands. Sometimes high fever indicates the dangerous condition of the patient. Occasionally an eruption appears which resembles the scarlatina rash.

Domfin litre dil. alt. *Scrof. 1* second dil. (diluted in milk) a teasponful every 5 minutes. At the commencement warm compresses of *Domfin*. Warm sprays of *Domfin* to the throat. Ointment of *Domfin* alt. with *Lin.* Gargles of *Domfin*, *Scrof. 1*, *Ang. 3* or *Red* El. Compress of *Feb. 2* to 24. Warm Baths of *Scrof. 5*, *Ang. 3* or *Canc. 5*. If there is much fever give *Feb. 1* in third dil. alternately with the other remedies. Applications of *Red*, *White*, or *Blue* El. If there is much vomiting or nausea give 3 globs. *Scrof. Giap.* dry on the tongue.

The room should be kept at 60° to 68° temperature but should be well ventilated, the patient being carefully protected from draughts. A kettle should be kept steaming in the room. Milk or egg flip should be given in teaspoonfuls or nutrient enemata should be administered.

Attendants should be particularly careful to avoid kissing the patient.

In this and other serious diseases medical assistance should be sought.

Diplopia : (See Eyes.)

Dipsomania : The patient must be kept from having access to alcoholic beverages and treated with *Ang. 1* in second dil. alt. *Scrof. 1* in third dil. A dry glob. of *Feb. 1* may be given each hour and *Feb. 2* ointment applied to 24.

Dislocation: The bone must first be carefully re-set. Afterwards *Ang. 1* or *Scrof. 1* alt *Canc. 1* or *3* with application of *Red* or *Blue* El. will hasten the cure.

Dizziness: (See Vertigo.)

Dropsy: an accumulation of serous fluid in the tissues immediately below the skin or in a serous cavity. It may be general or local. The former kind usually results from albuminuria, or cardiac disease, especially tricuspid regurgitation. The latter kind has generally a local cause.

Treatment—General Dropsy—*Feb. 1*, second dil. alt. *Scrof. 1*, second dil. At meals 3 globs. *Ang. 3*. Night and morning 3 dry globs. of *Canc. 2*. Apply *Red*, *Yellow* and *Blue* El. to 5, 18, 17. *Canc. 5* ointment to kidney region and *Feb. 2* to 24. Baths of *Canc. 5*.

A skilful Matteist says that *Scrof. 2* in the pint dilution alt. with *Canc. 2* in the quart dil., and *Ang. 2* in the two-quart dil., and 2 globs. *Feb. 1* in a little water at night have been found effectually to reduce dropsy.

For *Dropsy of Abdòmen*—*Feb. 1*, second dil. alt. *Canc. 2*, third dil. Apply compress of *Feb. 2* to 24. Ointment of *Canc. 5* to kidney region, and *White* El. to 5, 17, 18. Should *Canc. 2* not afford relief alternate with it *Ang. 3*, *2* or *1* in third dil., especially if the heart is affected, and apply *Blue* El. to heart. Sometimes *Canc. 3* or *5* are useful in lieu of *Canc. 2*.

In *Dropsy of Chest*, with difficulty of breathing, *Scrof. 1*, second dil. alt. *Pett. 1*, second dil. Apply *Red* alt. *Yellow* El. to 5, 18, and back of neck.

In *Dropsy of the Heart* (Hydropericarditis) *Ang. 3*,

third dil., alt. *Feb. 1*, third dil. Compresses of *Feb. 2* to 24 and *Ang. 2* to heart. Light applications of *Blue* El. to heart.

Dropsy of the Liver (see Cirrhosis)—*Feb. 1* second or third dil., with *Feb. 2* ointment to 24 should be used for a few days. Afterwards 5 globs. *Canc. 5* dry night and morning with *Ang. 2*, second dil. alt. *Feb. 1*, second or third dil.

Dropsy of the Ovaries—*Canc. 2*, second dil., alt. *Ang. 2*, third dil. Compress or ointment of *Canc. 5* to ovaries. Ointment of *Lin.* or *Scrof. 3* on ovaries. *Red* El. to 6. *Scrof. 1* alt. *Lin.* at meals.

Dropsy of the Womb—*Canc. 2*, third dil.

Dropsy of the Testicles: *Canc. 1* or *2* in second dil. sometimes alt. with *Ang. 1* or *3*.

Drowning: For restoring the apparently drowned, 5 globs. *Scrof. 1* first dil., with applications of *Red* El. to 5 and 18, and of *Blue* El. to heart. Rub the extremities with *White* El. Artificial respiration must be persistently used, care being taken to avoid pressure on the stomach, and friction of the extremities kept up for some time.

Drunkenness: 10 grains of *Scrof. 1* dry on the tongue. Repeat the dose after one hour. To remove the consequences of intoxication take *Scrof. 1* first dil. or *Ang. 3* second dil., 1 glob. *Canc. 5* dry on tongue per hour. Apply *White* El, to 11, 5. Lightly apply *Blue* El. to the heart. Baths of *Canc. 5*. *Feb. 2* Ointment to 24.

Dumbness: Incapacity for uttering articulate sounds, sometimes due to deafness, sometimes resulting from lesion of the hypoglossal nerve, paralysis of the tongue, especially through lead poisoning, or great emotional disturbances, &c., frequently arising from intellectual disorders. *Scrof. 1* second dil. or *Canc. 1* second dil.; alt. *Ang. 2* second dil. if there is any circulatory disorder. *Red* alt. *Yellow* El. to 18, 17, 9, 13. *Scrof. 5* or *Canc. 5* ointment to head. Baths of *Lin.* or *White* El. Certain forms are quite incurable.

Dysentery: A febrile disease. There is inflammation of the solitary and tubular glands of the large intestine, frequently followed by ulceration. Stools at first are feculent. Afterwards they contain blood, slime, &c. There are often much feebleness, headache, shivering and insomnia. In some cases ulceration is accompanied by sloughing of the mucous membrane or even by gangrene. Enlargement of the mesenteric glands is generally present, and frequently there is also organic disease of the liver. In the more serious forms of the disease the following symptoms appear :—Chilliness, followed by feverishness, distressing thirst, rapid pulse, very frequent stools, painful straining, severe griping, abdominal tenderness, and a pinched and anxious expression. In the most unfavourable cases there are extreme nervous prostration, excessive intestinal hæmorrhage, hiccough, nausea, delirium, and a marked increase in the stools of putrescent and gangrenous products which resemble the washings of decomposing flesh. The appearance of the first symptoms of Dysentery should be followed by the use *Scrof. Giap.* or *Scrof. 1*, first or litre dil., with warm fomentations of *Scrof. 1*. *Canc 5* ointment to abdomen, and *Feb. 2* ointment to 24. *Red* alt. *Yellow* El. to 5, 6, 11, 17. As soon as there is any blood in the stools give *Ang. 1* third dil. alt *Scrof. 1* second dil., or *Scrof. Giap.* second dil., with 1 glob. *Scrof. 1* dry hourly.

Apply *Blue* El. to 6, and *Ang. 3* ointment to 27 (very gently).

In the event of the disease passing into the grave form, give *Feb. 1* third dil., alt. *Canc. 1* second or third dil. in small teaspoonfuls every 5 to 10 minutes, and 1 glob. *Scrof. 1* dry hourly; enemata of *Canc. 5*.

In chronic cases the patient should remove to a non-malarious climate, should avoid salt meats, should wear a compress of *Canc. 5* over the abdomen, and another over the anus. He should use digestible food, and take frequent warm whole-body baths medicated with *Feb. 2*, *Ang. 3*, or *Canc. 5*. During convalescence *Scrof. Giap.* should be taken at meals, and the litre dil. of *Scrof. 1* during the day.

Dysmenorrhœa: Difficult and painful menstruation. See Menstruation.

Dyspepsia (Indigestion): This common ailment may result from a number of different causes, such as: deficiency or excess of food, improper food, eating too quickly, imperfect mastication of food, excessive or defective action of the muscular tissues, nerve centres or connecting nerves of the gullet, stomach, or intestines, obstructions in the alimentary canal, defective teeth, or improper quantity of or composition of the secretions by means of which the food undergoes the requisite chemical changes. The last-named cause is frequently brought into operation through perverted nervous influence, or abnormal blood supply. Everything that debilitates, such as worry, excessive toil, grief, &c., tends to produce Dyspepsia. The symptoms of Dyspepsia include discomfort in the abdomen, and sometimes heartburn or colic. There often are furred tongue, loss of appetite, constipation, or diarrhœa, vomiting, flatulence, eructations of gas, foul taste or breath, headache, palpitation, drowsiness, diminished mental energy, troubled or dreamy sleep. The treatment depends upon the cause, as well as upon the patient's peculiar temperament. In simple acute Dyspepsia give 10 globs. *Scrof. 1* dry on the tongue, and then *Scrof. 1* litre or second dil.; *Red* El. to 6; *Feb. 2* compress or ointment to 24. If there is flatulence, alternate *Feb. 1* second dil. with *Scrof. 1.* 3 globs. *Scrof. 2* dry, followed in twenty minutes by 3 globs, *Ver. 1* dry, or *Ver.* alt. *Scrof. Giap.* If there is any indication of biliousness, *Scrof. 5* must be substituted for *Scrof. 1.*

If the liver is affected and causes the Dyspepsia, take *Feb. 1* second dil., and apply *Feb. 2* compress and ointment to 24. If the circulation is at fault take *Ang. 1* second or third dil., and apply a compress of *Ang. 3* to the heart.

Dysphagia (difficulty of swallowing): This may arise from acute catarrh of the pharynx, tonsillitis, ulceration of the throat, laryngitis, laryngeal polypi, specific diseases which affect the throat, post-dipththeritic paralysis, hysterical affections, &c. Treatment depends upon the cause. Warm sprays of *Scrof. 1* or of *White* El. will be useful in some cases. If the affection is of a purely nervous character apply *White* El. with *Canc. 5.*

Ear: The ear is divided into three parts. There is first the external ear, including that concave part which projects from the side of the head, and the auditory canal which extends from this as far as the drum of the ear, a membrane which receives the waves of sound which pass

neighbouring nerve centres, and use third dilutions instead of first.

2. Otorrhœa : Discharge from the ear, usually purulent. Usually follows an ordinary cold and commonest in scrofulous children.

3. Otitis Media Purulenta : *Scrof. 1* or *5*, second or third dil. alt. *Canc. 1*, second or third dil., 5 globs. *Scrof. 5* at meals. Warm injections of *White* El. and water (30 drops to a teaspoonful) and also of *Canc. 5*. Should there appear any fragments of bone or cartilage in the discharge it may be known that there is caries of the bony canal. It will then be needful to give *Canc. 1* in second or third dil., with injections of *Canc. 1* alt. *Canc. 5*, while there are any signs of caries. Afterwards the foregoing treatment may be resumed.

4. Otalgia. Pain in ear ; Ear-ache. Treated like Otitis.

5. Buzzing in the ears Treat like Otitis, unless it arises from congestion, in patients with florid face and liable to throbbing headaches, when it will require 3 to 5 drops of *Blue* El. on sugar and application of *Blue* El. to 18, 17, the root of the ear (with the mouth open) and the muscles behind the ear.

6. Hæmorrhage from the Ear : *Ang. 2* or *1*, second dil., with *Canc. 5*, if it recurs frequently. Compress of *Ang. 3* to the ear and *Ang. 2* or *1* to the heart. Application of *Blue* El. to 18, 17, and very slightly over heart. *Ang. 3* ointment to back of ear.

III.—The Internal Ear. The auditory nerve may lose its function through hereditary syphilis. Partial deafness begins at from 5 to 15 years of age, and proceeds to total deafness. Treat as for Hereditary Syphilis.

Ecchymosis of Eyes: Extravasation of blood into the cellular tissues around the eye. (Black Eye): *Ang. 1*, second or third dil. Compress of *Blue* or *White* El. Ointment of *Ang. 3*. *Marina* lotion. Application of *Blue* El. to 1, 2.

Ecthyma: Pimples or pustules about the size of split peas, situated on elevated, reddened and indurated bases. They may be produced by any kind of irritant. *Scrof. 1* or *5* in second or third dil., with lotions and baths of *Canc. 1* or *5* alt. *Ang. 3*. Ointment of *Canc. 5* alt. *Ang. 3*.

Eczema (Psora): An acute or chronic inflammation of the skin, chiefly caused by the presence of excess of blood in a part as a result of local irritation, or of disturbed nervous function. Malassimilation, by acting as a disturber of nutrition and circulation of the skin, forms a predisposing cause. Eczema is non-contagious. It is accompanied by heat, itching, redness, slight swelling, and exudation. A crust forms which afterwards falls off. In some cases the exudation is considerable. Infantile eczema is sometimes complicated with bronchitis, and in this case it often happens that the inflammation of the surface membrane grows less when the internal inflammation increases, and *vice versâ*. The crusta lactea or milk-crust of children is one of the several varieties of eczema. *Scrof. 5* or *1* second or third dil., or *Canc. 1* third dil. alt. *Ang. 3* third dil. 2 drops *White* El. night and morning. Bath or lotions of *Canc. 5* or *Scrof. 1* alt. *Ang. 3*. Apply *Red* alt. *Yellow* El. to 5, 18, 17. Ointment of *Canc. 5* to 24. Compress of *White* El. In chronic cases of long standing, *Scrof. 1* quart dil., alt. *Feb. 1* quart dil., alt. *Ang. 1* two quart dil. *Scrof. 5* ointment is useful in some cases.

Elephantiasis Arabum: A disease which is endemic in India, China, Egypt, Arabia, &c., and which may be due to the presence in the blood of certain parasites. There are violent pains, fever, inflammation and hypertrophy of the integument and areolar tissue, especially of some part of the extremities and genital organs. Enormous scrotal or labial tumours sometimes appear, and the lower limbs frequently become like the legs of elephants. To combat febrile symptoms take *Feb. 1*, second or third dil., and apply *Feb. 2* in compress and ointment to 24. For the swellings of the blood vessels and lymphatics take *Canc. 4 or 1* alt. *Ang. 3* or *2*, with 5 globs. of *Scrof.* or *Scrof. 2* at each meal, and 3 to 5 globs. of *Scrof. 1* or *Lin.* dry on the tongue night and morning. Compress of *Canc. 5*, *Scrof. 5*, *Feb. 2*, *Green* or *Red* El. Ointments of *Canc. 5*. *Ang. 3*, *Scrof. 5*, *Lin.*, with *Ang. 3* to 27 and *Feb. 2* to 24. Apply *Red* alt. *Yellow* El. to corresponding nerves according to laws of polarity and to six chief points. Baths of *Ang. 3* alt. *Canc. 5*, *Lin.*, or *Scrof. 5*.

Emphysema: The distension of the spaces of the areolar tissue with air or any other gas. It may result from a wound of the lung, from rupture of the air vesicles during a violent expiratory effort, and from other causes. Subcutaneous Emphysema, as a rule, requires no treatment, but in very serious cases may be relieved by making a few punctures in the swelling with a triangular needle. Emphysema of the *lungs*, however, calls for very careful treatment, especially when it involves the whole of a lobe or the whole of one or both lungs. Its presence is marked by constant and growing difficulty in breathing and a smothering sensation in the chest. As the disease progresses the countenance becomes dusky and puffy, and the voice becomes feeble. The size of the chest increases, especially in its upper part. The disease is frequently complicated with Asthma, Bronchitis, Pleurisy, or Heart Disease. *Ang. 1*, third dil., alt *Canc. 1*, third dil.; 3 to 5 globs. of *Scrof. 1* at meals. Application of *Red* alt. *Yellow* El. to related nerves.

Enteralgia : Paroxysmal intestinal colic. A massive dose of *Scrof. 1* (5 to 10 globs. dry on the tongue) and the application of *White* El. to 12 should be followed by the use of *Scrof. 1*, second dil.

Enteritis : Inflammation of the intestines, which may be acute or chronic, local or general. It is caused by irritation. The symptoms vary. In mild cases there is an uneasiness over the abdomen, with colicky and griping pains, formation of gas, frequent stools and sometimes slight feverishness. In severe cases there is frequently high fever, much localised pain and tenderness, nausea, and thirst. Diarrhœa is present in the majority of cases. In the most serious forms of the disease there is often extreme prostration, leading on to complete collapse which, in the case of infants, is often rapidly fatal. Hiccough is frequently distressing. In chronic cases the patient becomes emaciated and the complexion assumes a muddy appearance. At the outset give 5 globs. of *Scrof 1* or *Scrof. Giap.* dry once an hour for six hours. If this does not check the attack give *Scrof. 1*, first dil., in frequent teaspoonfuls, for six hours. Then, if necessary, give 5 globs. *Ang. 3* night and morning, with *Scrof. 1*, second dil., alt. *Feb. 1* or *2* in dil. during the day. Apply *Canc. 5* ointment on abdomen. In obstinate cases give *Canc. 1*, *Ang. 3* and

Feb. 1, all in second dil., and a dry glob. of *Scrof. 1* once an hour, and apply *Feb. 2* ointment to 24. Should the resistance continue give *Canc. 5*, second or third dil.

Particular attention must be paid to diet. In a simple case as little food as possible should be given for a few hours. Even complete abstinence from food for 24 to 48 hours has been recommended. Milk and soda or lime water are most useful.

Epidemics: During the prevalence of these *Scrof. Giap.* should be taken as a prophylactic or preventive in doses of 3 to 5 globs. dry, twice daily. Special attention should be paid to the cleanliness of the person, to the sanitary state of the house, and to the diet. Over-fatigue and improper food should be avoided. Try to check at once any slight cold or other ailment.

Epilepsy: Spasmodic fits and loss of consciousness arising from increased irritability of some portion or portions of the nervous system. There may be an inherited tendency to them. Epilepsy may be caused by an alteration in the condition or action of the brain or its membranes in consequence of an attack of typhoid fever, scarlatina, &c. Other causes include injuries of the trunk, limbs, or viscera, alteration of the quantity or quality of blood, irritation of the sexual organs brought on by self-abuse and worms.

Treatment must be most cautiously administered. No stronger dilution than the third must on any account be used and only 6 to 10 teaspoonfuls of this should be taken daily. In one case, when the first dilution was used the number of fits was increased. The remedy taken must harmonise with the suspected cause. If the circulation is at fault use *Ang. 3, 2* or *1*, third dil. If worms, *Ver. 1*, third dil. If the condition of the brain or its membrane, or of any part of the absorbent system is at fault give *Scrof. 1* or *Canc. 1*, third dil., alt. *Ang. 1*, third dil.

Epistaxis: Bleeding from the nose. Sometimes occasioned by violent sneezing or coughing, especially in persons with a hæmorrhagic tendency. It often happens in boys about the age of puberty, and in girls as a form of vicarious menstruation. Sometimes it occurs as a relief to determination of blood to the head, or in connection with heart disease, dropsy, &c. *Ang. 3, 2* or *1* in third dil. 3 drops of *Blue* El. on sugar. Repeat at the expiration of an hour. Syringe the nostrils with *Ang. 3* or *2*, and apply compress of the same remedy to the heart. *Blue* El. to base of nose, 18, 17, and forehead.

Eruptions: Treat like Eczema. But when it is desired to bring out suppressed eruptions give strong doses of *Scrof. 1*, first dilution.

Erysipelas: an inflammation of the integument, lymphatic vessels and lymph-spaces, which not only tends to spread through the body, but may also infect other individuals. In simple cutaneous erysipelas there are chilliness, loss of appetite, malaise, nausea, and a temperature of at least 103° fahrenheit. Within 24 hours a part of the skin becomes inflamed and bright red in colour. The inflammation spreads. Sometimes small vesicles arise which ordinarily contain clear yellow serum. The pulse is rapid and feeble. After the inflammation has subsided the cuticle falls off, and sometimes the neighbouring glands suppurate. Sometimes erysipelas affects the mucous membrane of the pharynx and larynx. In serious cases there are high fever, violent delirium and excessive diarrhœa. At the onset apply *Red* El. to 18, and give 5 globs. *Scrof. 1* or *Scrof. 5* dry on the tongue. Then persist with *Scrof. 1* or *5*, second dil., or, in mixed or sanguine temperaments, *Scrof. 1* alt. *Ang. 1*, second dil. Apply warm compress of *White* El. to the affected part. Hot baths of *Canc. 5*. To allay fever give *Feb. 1*, second dil. Nourishing diet is necessary but no solid meat food must be taken. In Phlegmonous Erysipelas, there is great swelling, the spaces in the areolar tissue become filled with a serous fluid which gradually becomes turbid. In a few days the greater part of a limb may be involved. Occasionally there are ulcerations and moist gangrene. *Ang. 1*, second dil. Compress *White* or *Blue* El. Apply *Feb. 2* to 24. To check the return of Erysipelas *Feb. 1*, second dil., may be given to persons of bilious temperament who have a natural predisposition to the disease.

Erythema : a redness of the skin, which disappears on pressure but reappears when this is removed. There is sometimes a slight itching. *Scrof. 1*, second or third dil. or *Canc. 1*, second or third dil. If there are any feverish symptoms give also *Feb. 1*, second or third dil.

Excrescences : Bony, Fleshy, Gangrenous, Scrofulous, Syphilitic. See Scrofula, Syphilis, and Tumours. In cases which do not come under these three heads give *Scrof. 1* or *5*, litre dil., or *Canc. 1*, litre dil., and apply compresses of *Canc. 5* alt. *Scrof. 1* alt. *Ang. 3*. Also baths of *Scrof. 5*. In fleshy excrescences apply compress of *Blue* El.

Exhaustion : *Scrof. 1*, litre dil. Drops of *White* El.

Exophthalmic Goitre : See Graves' Disease.

Exostosis: a bony outgrowth resulting from cancer, scrofula, or syphilis. *Scrof. 1*, third or second dil., or *Scrof. 2*, third dil., alt. *Canc. 4*, third dil., with *Ven.*, third dil. if syphilitic origin is suspected. Globs. of *Canc. 4* and *Scrof. 1* at meals. Baths of *Canc. 5*. Applications of *Blue* El. to related nerves and *Red* to 18. Compress of *Canc 5*. *Feb. 2* ointment to 24.

Eye: The point of the eyeball is covered with a mucous membrane called the *conjunctiva* which also lines the inner surfaces of the eyelids. Beneath this is the *cornea*, a transparent horny coat. Next comes an *aqueous chamber* at whose base are the *iris* and the *pupil*, the former of which gives the colour to the eye. Behind the iris is the *crystalline lens* through which the rays of light pass into the vitreous humour which occupies the greater part of the eyeball. At the back of this vitreous chamber is the *retina* which is from $\frac{1}{50}$th to $\frac{1}{200}$th of an inch thick and is formed by the expansion of the fibres of the optic nerve which carries the vibrations to the brain. Binding the whole together is the *sclerotic coat* or tunic of the eye. As each part of this complex organ is liable to disease, it would require considerable space to indicate the treatment. A few hints only can be given. It should be noted, however, that *Marina* and *Scrofoloso*, used internally and externally are of special value in eye diseases, and that *White*, *Red* or *Blue* El. applied to 1, 2, 3, 17 are exceedingly valuable adjuncts.

(1) Inflammation of the *conjunctiva* (conjunctivitis). *Scrof. 1*, third dil. alt. *Mar.* third dil. *Ang. 3* ointment at night over the sub-orbital and super-orbital region. *Mar.* lotion may be applied by means of a saturated strip of

lint laid from temple to temple. This must not be covered or left on when dry.

(2) *Amaurosis*: Blindness resulting from white atrophy of the optic nerve, due to syphilis or tobacco-smoking, or the pressure of tumours, &c., upon the nerve. *Scrof. 1* or *2*, third dil. alt. *Ang. 1* third dil. alt. *Mar.* third dil. Eye baths of *Mar.* with warm water. *White*, *Red* or *Red* alt. *Yellow* El. to 1, 2, 3, 17, forehead, *White* or *Blue* to centre of cranium. If syphilitic origin is suspected, give *Ven.* second dil. If there is cerebral congestion give *Scrof. 2* second dil. alt. *Ang. 3*, second dil. Apply comp. of *Scrof.* alt. *Ang.*

(3) *Amblyopia*: obscurity of vision. Treat as amaurosis and use baths of *Canc. 5*, *Ang. 3*, *Scrof.* or *White* El. with comp. to entire head of *White* El. or *Canc. 5*.

(4) *Bleared Eyes*: Treat as No. 3. Also comp. on closed eye with *Ang. 3*, *2* or *1*, or *White* or *Blue* El.

(5) *Cataract*: an opacity of part or whole of the crystalline lens, varying from milky to chalky white. *Scrof. 1* second or third dil. alt. *Ang. 3*, third dil. alt. *Mar.* third dil. Apply *Scrof. 1* and *Ang. 3* externally in comp. and *Red* El. to 2, 3. Baths of *Canc. 5*, *Scrof. 5*, *Ang. 3*. Ointment of these three remedies to the head and of *Feb. 2* and *Canc. 5* to 24. When the cataract begins to disperse take care to shade the eye from the light.

(6) *Choroiditis*: Treat like Keratitis. If syphilitic origin is suspected treat the constitutional disease.

(7) *Diplopia*: Double vision. Squinting. Strabismus. This may be convergent, divergent, or there may be an upward or downward divergence between the direction of vision of tne two eyes. It may be owing to paralysis or

to paresis of the nerve of one eye, to excessive development of both the muscles which turn the front of the eyes inward, or to defective vision of the squinting eye. In those cases which are amenable to treatment: *Ang. 3* or *1* third dil. or *Ang. 3* third dil. alt. *Scrof. 1* third dil. and *Mar.* third dil., comp. of *Mar.*, *Green* El. over eyes, and of *Canc. 5*, *Scrof. 5*, *Ang. 2*. *Red* alt. *Yellow* to 3, 17, 1, 2. Eye-baths of *Mar.*

(8) *Ecchymosis*: See the word.

(9) *Hæmorrhage*: Sometimes a sign of nocturnal epilepsy or of hæmorrhage within the cranium. *Ang. 1* or *3*, third dil. *Blue* El. to 18, 17, and nerves of head; *Ang. 3* alt. *Canc. 5* ointment to head and *Feb. 2* alt. *Canc. 5* to to 24.

(10) *Indistinct Vision*: *Mar.* third dil. and *Red* El. to 1, 2 and 3 will suit some cases. But an effort must be made to ascertain cause and treat accordingly.

(11) *Iritis*: Inflammation of the Iris. Treat like Keratitis, taking care not to omit *Ven.* third dil. if the disease is of syphilitic origin.

(12) *Keratitis*: Inflammation of the Cornea. In the suppurative form use *Scrof. 1*, third dil. alt. *Mar.* third dil. In the vascular form *Ang. 3*, third dil. alt. *Mar.*; and in the interstitial form alternate these remedies with *Ven.* third dil.

(13) *Ophthalmia*: Forms of inflammation originating in the superficial structures of the eye. They include catarrhal, contagious, granular, infantile, simple, vascular, venereal and rheumatic. Treatment as in Conjunctivis (which is a form of ophthalmia) adding *Ven.* second or third dil. in cases of syphilitic origin. In cases of purulent

ophthalmia *Scrof. 1* third dil. and *Canc. 1* third dil. may be given.

(14) *Photophobia*: Intolerance of light, occurring in all inflammatory eye diseases, and also in cerebral irritation, meningitis, &c. In many of the first class of cases this has been successfully treated with *Red* El. or *Red* alt. *Yellow* El. to 1, 2, 18, 17; comp. of *White* El. and *Canc. 5* ointment to whole head.

(15) *Retinitis*: Treat like Keratitis.

(16) *Sclerotitis*: Treat like Keratitis.

(17) *Shortsightedness*: Apply *Red* El. to 2, 3.

(18) *Staphyloma*: a protusion of the sclerotic or of the cornea. *Scrof. 1* third dil. alt. *Ang. 3, Mar.* In cases arising from syphilis add *Ven.*, third dil.

(19) *Strabismus*: See Diplopia.

(20) *Specks in Cornea*: See Interstitial Keratitis.

(21) *Ulceration of Cornea*: Treat as Ophthalmia (purulent.)

Eyelids, *Inflammation of*: *Scrof. 1* second dil. or *Canc. 1* second dil. alt. *Ang. 1*, second dil.; Comp. of *Scrof. 1* or *Canc. 5* alt. *Ang. 3* or of *White* El. Apply *Blue* or *Red* alt. *Yellow* El. to 5, 18, 1, 2, 3 and forehead.

Paralysis of: Treat as above and also apply *Red* El. comp. to eyelids.

Spasms of, with Vertigo: *Ang. 2, 3* or *1*, second dil. alt. *Canc. 2*, with comp. of *Ang. 3* to 2 and 3, and application of *White* El. to 5, 18, 2.

Face, Blemishes on the: Wash with *Acqua per la pelle*. If resulting from a disordered liver take *Feb. 1* litre dil. Apply ointment or compress of *Feb. 2* or *1*, or *Canc. 5* to 24, and *Red* alt. *Yellow* El. to the facial nerves.

Impetigo: See Impetigo.

Lupus: See Lupus.

Pains in the (congestive): *Ang. 1* second dil. or *Ang. 2* second or third dil.; *Canc. 5* or *Ang. 2* ointment to head; Compress of *Ang. 3*, *Ang.* or *Ang. 2* to heart.

Pains in the (rheumatic): *Ang. 1* second dil. alt. *Scrof. 5* litre dil.; *Red* alt. *Yellow* to heart; ointment of *Canc. 5*, *Scrof.*, *Scrof. 5*; compress or baths of *Canc.* 5.

Fainting Fit (Syncope): Suspended animation consequent on failure of the heart's action. This may be due to fatty degeneration of the heart, compression of the heart by tight-fitting clothes, extreme heat, concussion of the brain, shocks to the nervous system, hæmorrhage, &c. The patient should be placed on his back, and his dress loosened. The windows of the room should be opened so that he may breathe pure air. 10 globules of *Scrof. 1* should be placed upon his tongue and afterwards a few doses of *Scrof. 1* first dil. should be given. *Red* El. should be applied to 6, 11, 18, 17.

Falling of Bowels, Womb &c.: See Prolapsus.

Falling Sickness: See Epilepsy.

Favus (Tinea favosa): a disease which usually affects the scalp and is characterised by the appearance of circular copper-coloured crusts which are penetrated by the hair. Long treatment is often needed with *Scrof. 1* second or third dil.; comp. of *Lin.*, *Canc. 5*, *Scrof. 5* or *White* El. Should this not be sufficient alt. *Canc. 1* or *Ang. 3* with *Scrof. 5*, *2* or *1*.

Feet, *Contusion of*: *Feb. 1*, second dil. alt. *Canc. 1*, second dil.; Comp. of *Red* El.

Sprain: Comp. of *Red* El.

Sweating: *Scrof. 1*, litre dil. alt. *Ang. 3*, second dil. Apply *Red* alt. *Yellow* El. to 5, 18, 17, 6, 7; also *Red* El. to 8, and *Yellow* El. to 14. Baths of *Canc. 5*, *Scrof. 1* or *Ang. 2*.

Pain in: *Feb. 1*, litre dil. alt. *Canc. 1* second dil.

Fevers: If it be true, as Dr. Broadbent declares it is, that "every school in every age has had its theory of the febrile process," the author may be pardoned if he declines to commit himself to any. It must suffice to indicate what are the essential phenomena and symptoms of fevers. These include (1) a rise of temperature; (2) increase in the rapidity of the pulse; (3) modifications of the secretions and excretions; (4) disordered respiration, which is generally increased in frequency; (5) increased combustion of the tissues; (6) disturbance of the nervous system. The last is specially noticeable in the invasive stage, and is marked by rigors, headache, &c. Afterwards there frequently is delirium. It is thought by some that it is because the nerve tension is diminished and the usual check to oxidation consequently withdrawn, that tissue change proceeds at a more rapid rate and a higher temperature is produced. They believe that the sympathetic and pneumogástric nerves are specially involved. In the treatment of fever, *Feb. 1* in dil. and *White* El. in drops, with *Feb. 2* ointment and comp. to 24 are most generally useful. Sometimes a few teaspoonfuls of *Feb. 2.* in first dil. subdue fever with marvellous rapidity. Use also fever pack. The following are the chief fevers:

Dandy Fever (Dengue): characterised by severe continuous pains in the head and eyeballs, joints and muscles, great weakness, scarlet rash, irritation of the skin, sore throat. Its invasion is generally sudden. Pulse is rapid, (102 to 140) and temperature is high (103° or even 105°). In its malignant form it is known as black fever. *Feb. 1* second or third dil. In dangerous cases give also a few teaspoonfuls of *Ang. 3* second or third dil. per diem. *Feb. 2* compress; *Feb. 2* ointment to 24.

Intermittent Fever: resulting from the introduction of a malarial baccillus into the body. There are enlargement of the spleen and congestion of the liver. The fever is paroxysmal. In each paroxysm there are three stages: (1) The cold stage. The limbs feel cold, and the back of the body becomes chilly. The teeth chatter and the whole frame shivers. (2) The hot stage, with throbbing headaches, burning dry skin, flushed face and sparkling eyes. Temperature rises to 105°, 107° or even higher. (3) The sweating stage, during which the perspiration pours out in considerable quantities. The varying intervals between the paroxysms give the names to the different types of the fever, *e.g.* Quotidian, with daily paroxysms; Tertian, with fits on alternate days, &c. Before the paroxysms *Feb. 1*, first dil., a dessertspoonful every hour; *Feb. 2* comp. and ointment to 24. During the paroxysm *Feb. 1* second dil., a teaspoonful every five minutes, and *Feb. 2* compress to 24. These must be renewed as soon as they are dry. A wet pack, a vapour bath, or a blanket bath would be useful. A *Feb. 2* compress should be worn continually. At the end of a week if there is no improvement give *Feb. 1* litre dil. a teaspoonful every half hour. In the pernicious form of the fever *Feb. 1* should be given every half-hour in second dil. (tablespoonful doses) in the intervals, and the same remedy in small teaspoonfuls during the fits. Avoid stimulants.

Febricula : Simple fever of one or two days' duration. *Feb. 1*, second dil., *Feb. 2* ointment and comp. to 24; *Canc. 5* ointment to kidney region. Give a wet pack or blanket bath. Wear a fever compress.

Malarial (Marsh miasm) : a fever which results from the action upon the nervous system of a poison which ordinarily emanates from moist soils more or less rich in organic matter, and which is not brought under cultivation. Treatment as in Febricula.

Miliary : a febrile condition attended with the eruption of vesicles in the skin. *Feb. 1* second dil., alt. *Scrof. 1*, second dil. Tepid baths of *Feb. 2*.

Milk Fever: The patient is seized with a shivering fit. It seems as if cold water were running down her spine. The breast becomes swollen and sensitive. Then follow intense headaches, and pains in the limbs. *Feb. 1* second dil.; *Feb. 2* to 24.

Puerperal: a continued fever often resulting from the absorption of septic matter, and occurring after child-birth. It is contagious. It is generally a rapidly fatal disease. *Feb. 1* second dil. alt. *Canc. 1*, second dil. *Canc. 5* ointment or compress to abdomen.

Relapsing : A very infectious fever resembling typhus. The invasion is very sudden and is generally ushered in with a severe rigor, sharp frontal headaches, giddiness and pains in the back and limbs. In children, the disease sometimes begins with a heavy sleep. There are vomiting tendencies, pains over the stomach, liver and spleen, great thirst, rapid pulse, and febrile urine. The temperature rises to 104°, 105°, or even 108°. The crisis is accompanied by profuse perspiration. A few days after the symptoms have disappeared there is a sudden relapse which lasts from a few hours to a week. Other relapses sometimes follow. Treat like Typhus.

Remittent: Malarial fevers may be of a remittent type. They are then more dangerous than in their other form. In the hot stage there are obstinate vomiting, a very rapid pulse, quick respiration, and an anxious countenance, In the morning there is a remission which lasts from two to twelve hours and is followed by the distressing hot stage. *Feb. 1* second or third dil. *Feb. 2* ointment and compress.

Rheumatic. Acute Rheumatism: At first there are soreness and stiffness, aching pains in the limbs and trunk, articular pains, sore throat and chilliness. Then the patient feels severe pain in at least one of his joints, he experiences a shivering fit and his temperature rapidly rises. His face and body becomes bedewed with sour acrid perspiration. His joints swell and become tender. His pulse is frequent and he devotes all his thought to keeping his joints in the most easy position possible. His tongue is covered with a thick, white, moist fur, and his mouth is parched. In many cases his heart also is affected. The temperature rises to from 100° to 107°, but in fatal forms the temperature has been known to rise to 110° or higher. *Scrof. 1*, first and second dil. alt. *Ang. 3* second or third dil.; *Green* El. to the joints; *Scrof. 5* or *Canc. 5* ointment or oil for joints. *Feb. 2* ointment to 24, and *Ang. 3* to heart. The patient should be clothed in flannel and kept in a comfortable bed. A blanket bath or cool wet pack may be administered. Or a vapour bath may be tried. The feet and hands should be kept in hot mustard and water. Great care must be taken to avoid chills. It is a good plan to wrap up the joints in cotton wool.

Scarlet Fever: Commences with chilliness and rapid rise of temperature. Face becomes flushed. There are marked sore throat, vomiting, frequent strong and full pulse, and strawberry-like tongue. On the second day minute eruptions appear on the neck and upper part of the chest, which coalesce to form patches. The rash reaches its height on the 4th or 5th day; then gradually fades. The skin peels off. Temperature reaches 104° to 106°. *Feb. 1*, second dil. alt. *Scrof. 1* second or third dil., a teaspoonful every 5 minutes. *White* El. to 18; *Feb. 2* compress to 24; hot baths of *Canc. 5*, 2 drops *White* El. twice a day. In obstinate cases add *Canc. 1*, second dil. Hot baths and wet packs are useful in most cases. A fever compress should be worn, and changed when dry.

Typhoid: At first there is persistent diarrhœa. Then follow marked frontal headache, pain and tenderness in the abdomen, and enlarged spleen. On the 7th to the 12th day appears a rash composed of minute slightly raised rose-coloured spots. The temperature rises 2° each morning, but falls 1° each evening. It reaches at last from 104° to 106° and then gradually descends. *Feb. 1* third dil. in teaspoonfuls every five or ten minutes alt. *Scrof. 1* second dil. Those who understand hydropathy should use a fomenting pack, which is most potent in arresting the progress of the disease. During first and second stage *Feb. 2* or *Canc. 5* ointment to 24; *Canc. 5* baths. The remedy may also be administered in milk. Apply *Red* alt. *Yellow* El. to 5, 17, 18. In the third or dynamic stage, where recovery is well-nigh despaired of, give 1 glob. *Canc. 5* hourly, and apply *Canc. 5* ointment on abdomen, and apply *White* or *Red* El. to 5. 17, 18, dorsal spine and soles of feet. During convalesence give *Scrof. 1* as a tonic.

Typhus: The onset of this disease speedily produces prostration. The patient's countenance becomes muddy and there is a dusky flush on the cheeks. Low nervous symptoms appear. On the fourth or fifth day irregular dusky red mottling and mulberry spots are seen about the back of the wrists, or on the epigastrium. These spread over the entire body. The skin gives off a peculiar odour. The temperature rises without any intermission up to 105°. The fever lasts from 14 to 21 days. Treatment as in Typhoid.

Yellow Fever: a contagious continuous fever. Its invasion is sudden, with intense headache, rigors, pain in the limbs and back, and rapid rise of temperature to from 102° to 110°. The pulse does not rise proportionately. There are congestion of the conjunctiva, skin, &c. The tongue is red at the tip and coated with thick yellow fur at the centre and root. In most cases there is vomiting of altered blood from the stomach. *Feb. 1* second or third dil.; *Feb. 2* ointment and compress to 24; *Canc. 5* ointment to kidney region; 5 drops *White* El. every four hours. Warm and vapour baths are recommended by some. Light and nutritious diet and pure air are of the first importance.

Finger (Whitlow in): *Scrof.* litre dil.; ointment of *Canc. 5*. Compress of *Scrof. 1*, or of *Canc. 5* and *White* El.

Fistula: a narrow canal or pipe extending from a free surface to some seat of local irritation. In general:

Scrof., litre dil. alt. *Canc. 1* litre dil.; compress and baths of *Scrof. 1* or *Ang. 3.*

Fistula of anus: Take *Scrof. 1* litre dil. alt *Canc. 4* litre dil. Apply compress of *Canc. 5* alt. *Ang. 3.* Baths of *Canc. 5* or *Lin.*; *Red* alt. *Yellow* El.

Fistula of gums: Take *Canc. 4* litre dil. alt. *Ang. 2* litre dil. Apply *Canc. 5* ointment to the jaw. Use mouth washes of *Canc. 5*, *Canc. 4* or *White* El.

Fistula of lachrymal duct: a small ulceration formed in the canal belonging to the lachrymal or tear-forming apparatus: Take *Scrof. 1* first or second dil. alt. with *Canc. 1* or *4* second dil. Compress of *Scrof. 1* or of *Green* El. if there is suppuration. Apply *Red* El. to 2, 3, 17, 18.

Fistula of scrotum: Take *Scrof.* litre dil. alt. *Canc. 1*, *Canc. 4* or *Canc. 5* litre dil. Compress of *Canc.* 5, *Scrof. 1* or *Ang. 3*, with sitz-baths of same or of *Lin.*

Fistula stercoraceous (of right groin): *Scrof. 1* dil. alt. *Canc.* dil. Baths of *Canc. 5.*

Fits: See Ague, Apoplexy, Convulsions, Epilepsy, Fainting, Hysteria. For Epilepsy give *Ang. 3* third dil.

Flatulence: The undue generation of gases in the stomach and intestines results from functional derangement or nervous debility. Dissolve 1 globule of *Scrof. 1* or *5* in a half-pint of hot water and drink as warm as can be borne. Take 5 globules of *Scrof. 1* or *5* in the beverage at meals. Avoid starchy foods. Well rub *Feb. 2* ointment over the hypochondriac region and apply *Red* El, to the pit of the stomach twice a day.

Flea-bites: See Bites.

Fracture: To accelerate cure, after the surgeon has set the bone, take *Scrof. 1* in second dil. Apply *Red* or

Blue El. to corresponding nerves. Compress of *Blue* or *White* El. or of *Canc. 5* or *Scrof. 5* to the seat of the fracture.

Frost-bites: a local effect of extreme cold, and consequent contraction of the capillaries. The passage of red blood corpuscles is thus impeded and the tissues degenerate. *Ang. 1* or *2* litre dil. alt. *Scrof. 1* first dil. If the face is affected apply *Blue* El. to 17, 18, and compress of *Ang. 3* to face. Give 1 globule of *Canc. 5* hourly. For subsequent results of Frost-bites *Red* alt. *Yellow* El. to corresponding points. Baths *Scrof. 5* alt. *White* El.

Fungus Hæmatodes: Soft malignant growths which bleed easily. Treat like Cancer, but alternate *Scrof. 1* second dil. with the *Ang.* and *Canc.*

Furunculus: See Boils.

Galactorrhœa: See Milk, flow of.

Gall Stones: Concretions wholly or chiefly composed of cholesterin which are found in the biliary passages, gall bladder, cystic, common or hepatic duct. While they are in the gall bladder they seldom produce any painful symptoms, but on their passage thence they first cause dull pain, then vomiting, rigors, feverishness, intense shooting and burning pains in the right hypochondrium, which sometimes extend as far as the right shoulders. There is tenderness over the region of the liver. Jaundice is common. The calculi are expelled with the stools. *Scrof. 1* or *2* first dil. alt. *Feb. 1* second dil., 5 globules of same remedies at meals; 5 globules *Feb. 1* dry on the tongue on waking; *Feb. 2* ointment to 24; baths of *Scrof. 5* alt. *Feb. 2*; compress of *Feb. 2* (10 globules) alt. *Canc. 5* (20 globules).

Ganglion: a cystic tumour near a tendon or a chronic dropsical swelling in the common sheath of a group of tendons. *Canc. 1* second dil. alt. *Ang. 3* second dil.; 5 globules *Scrof.* at meals; compress of *Canc. 1* or *5*, *Lin.* or *White* El.; *Lin.* or *Canc. 5* ointment; *Red* alt. *Yellow* to corresponding nerves.

Gangrene: mortification of a part of the tissues similar to that which takes place throughout the body at death. *Canc. 1* first or second dil. alt. *Ang. 3* first dil.; warm compress of *Canc. 5*; *White* or *Green* El. (the latter after operations); applications of *White* or *Red* El. alt. *Yellow* El. to corresponding nerves. *Canc. 5* baths are sometimes useful. Special efforts must be made to support the patient's strength by nourishing diet.

Gastralgia: Pain in the stomach: *Scrof. 1* first dil.; *White* or *Blue* El. to 6; *Feb. 2* ointment to 24.

Glandular Swellings: In general treat as in Ganglion. In scrofulous cases begin with *Scrof. 1* first dil. using *Canc. 1* second dil. when the swellings suppurate or when they are obstinate. Baths of *Scrof.* or *Canc. 5* alt. *Lin.* *Lin*, ointment.

Glaucoma: See Eye, Diseases of.

Gleet: *Ang. 3* second dil.; sitz-baths of *Ang. 3*. See also Blenorrhœa.

Gingivitis: Inflammation of the gums: *Scrof. 1* litre dil. or *Canc. 1* alt. *Ang. 3* litre dil. Wash the mouth with lotions of *Scrof. 1*.

Goitre: Enlargement of the gland situated near the thyroid or shield-like cartillage which forms the prominence known as Adam's apple. A disease prevalent in magnesium limestone districts such as Derbyshire. Hence its popular designation "Derbyshire neck." Take 5 globules of *Canc. 4* dry on the tongue twice a day, or 1 globule of *Canc. 5* dry hourly, second dil. of *Canc. 1* or of *Canc. 1* alt. *Scrof.* or *Ang. 3* second dil. Oil of *Canc. 5.* Ointment of *Ang. 3.* Compress of *White* or *Blue* El. or *Canc. 5.* *Red* alt. *Yellow* El. to corresponding nerves, and to base of gland.

Gonorrhœa: For the first four or five days give *Ang. 3.* When the inflammation has been reduced and the flux has begun, take *Ang. 3* or *Scrof. 1* alt. *Ven.* litre or second dil., 5 globules of *Scrof. 1* in beverage at meals, and 5 to 10 drops of *Yellow* El. once a day in a teaspoonful of water. Apply *Blue* El. or *Red* alt. *Yellow* El. to 18, 20, 22, 25. Injection of *Scrof.* alt. *Canc. 5.* A light and moderate diet, abstinence from alchoholic beverages, the use of a suspensory bandage and rest are recommended. Tepid baths of *Ang. 3.* After the flux has ceased, give *Scrof. 1,* first or litre dil.

Gout: a constitutional disease which is attributed to the presence in the system of an abnormal quantity of uric or lithic acid. This may result from special hereditary tendency; from the use of diet in which there is an excess of nitrogen, of alcoholic beverages, and especially of burgundy, madeira, sherry and marsala wines or of malt liquors; or from lead poisoning. The inflammation which occurs in an acute attack of articular gout is believed by some to result from nature's attempt to rid herself of the excess of uric acid. The gouty inflammation usually sets in around the smaller joints and most frequently around the metatarso-phalangeal joint of the great toe. It is often preceded by disorders of the digestive organs, nervous derangements, fretfulness, lowness of spirits, neuralgia, and the secretion of high-coloured urine. As a rule, the first paroxysm of pain comes on about 2 a.m. and is felt in the great toe or in some small joint in the foot or hand. The pain is so severe that sleep is prevented. It subsides during the day but recurs at night. There are symptoms of inflammation accompanied by considerable local heat. The attack lasts for a few days. Subsequent attacks may be expected, and chronic gouty inflammation is sometimes established. With this are frequently associated chronic catarrh, chronic skin diseases, or chronic cystitis. *Scrof. 1*, first dil., or if obstinate, *Scrof. 2* or *5*, litre dil. alt. *Ang. 2* or *3*, second dil. In chronic cases *Canc. 1*, second dil., and 5 globules of *Canc. 5* in the morning, 5 globules of *Scrof. 5* in beverage at meals twice daily. Compress of cotton wool medicated with *Canc. 5*, *Scrof. 1*, *Scrof. 5*, *White* or *Green* El. to the affected joints, 3 drops *Blue* El. once a day if the heart is not affected. Application of *Red* alt. *Yellow* El. to 5, 17, 18, and painful nerves. Ointment of *Canc. 5*, *Lin.*, *Scrof. 1* or *Scrof. 5* to the seat of the disease, and also of *Feb. 2* to 24. Baths of *Canc. 5* or *White* El. alt. *Ang. 3*. Take little if any animal food with nitrogenous vegetable food. Celery is strongly recommended by some practitioners, but this should not be taken with much salt, as this condiment should be avoided as much as possible. Total abstinence is helpful. Exercise is beneficial.

Gout, Rheumatic: a popular name for rheumatoid arthritis. Unlike true gout this complaint is not preceded by premonitory symptoms, the inflammation affects larger joints, and is less severe than in gout. The disease tends to involve joint after joint and often causes deformity. *Scrof. 1* or *2*, litre or second dil.; 5 globules *Scrof. 1* dry morning and evening, or in beverage at meals. Baths of *Canc. 5* or *Scrof.* *Feb. 2* ointment to 24. *Lin.* ointment to joints. Compress of *Canc. 5* to 24, of *Ang. 2* or *3* to heart, and friction of *Green* El. to affected joints. *Red* alt. *Yellow* El. to corresponding nerves and chief points. Baths of *Canc. 5* or *Lin.*

Gravel: Deposit of reddish brown crystals of lithic acid or other gritty particles in the urine. Treat with *Scrof. 1*, second dil. alt. *Ang. 2*, second dil., and with the other remedies prescribed under Calculus (renal).

Green Sickness: See Chlorosis.

Grippe: See Influenza.

Hæmatemesis: Vomiting of blood resulting from ulcer in the stomach, venous congestion, &c. It is generally preceded by a sensation of faintness and a feeling of weight at the pit of the stomach. When the amount of blood vomited has been large the patient should lie down and rest, and should abstain from taking food by the mouth. If needful for the support of strength nutrient enemata should be given. At the outset give 10 to 20 drops of *Blue* El. in a tablespoonful of water. Then *Ang. 3* or *2*, second dil.: a teaspoonful every 5 minutes. Apply *Red* El. to soles of feet. To prevent recurrence *Ang. 3* or *1*, litre dil. alt. *Canc. 1*, litre dil.

Hæmoptysis: spitting of blood, proceeding from the pulmonary artery or its radicles, the bronchial capillaries or the aorta or one of its branches. Sometimes there is only a slight tinging of the sputum. At other times as much as a quart or two of blood is brought up. In the latter case the patient is considerably prostrated by the attack. The medical treatment must be supplemented by absolute rest. Even speaking should be abstained from for a time. Stimulants must be avoided. The diet should be restricted to cold articles. 2 drops *Blue* El. once an hour. *Ang. 2*, second or third dil. alt. *Canc. 1*, second dil. Application of small compress of *Ang. 2* or of *Blue* El. to the heart. If the hæmorrhage comes from the respiratory tract alternate *Pet. 1*, second dil. with this.

Hæmorrhage : Bleeding from any part of the body, resulting from injury or from disease. Apply compress of *Blue* El. or of *Ang. 3*. Compress to heart of *Ang. 3*. Take *Ang. 1* or *2* in second dil.

Of womb : Treat as above and add sitz-baths of *Ang. 3*, and *Feb. 2* ointment to 24.

Hæmorrhoids : See Piles.

Hair, Falling of the : *Scrof. 5*. second dil. Compress or lotions of *Scrof. 5* or *Lin.* (the latter was found extremely useful by one lady). *Red* and *Yellow* El. to temples, 16, 17, 18. *Lin.* ointment. Baths of *Scrof. 5* alt. *Canc. 5*. Wash the head with *White* El. When the hair leaves white circular bald patches *Ven.* also must be taken internally and applied externally.

Hallucinations : Give *Feb. 1*, second dil. alt. *Canc. 1* second dil. Apply *Canc. 5* ointment to head and *Feb. 2* ointment to 24.

Hay Fever : Catarrh, affecting the mucous membrane of the eyes, nose, bronchi, &c., accompanied by difficulty of breathing. Due to the influence of pollen grains which float in the air during the summer. Persons subject to it should avoid districts where there is much hay-grass. At the outset take 5 to 8 globules of *Scrof. 1* dry on the tongue. Afterwards take *Scrof. 1*, third dil. A dry globule of *Pet. 1* may be given every hour or two.

Headache, or Cephalalgia: There are numerous varieties, originating in very different causes.

1. If due to disease of the brain, treatment must be directed to the removal of the cerebral affection, and *Canc. 5* ointment applied to the head.

2. If resulting from active congestion, in cases of hypertrophy of the left ventricle of the heart, irregular menstruation, &c., give *Ang. 3*, second or third dil. Apply compress *Ang. 3* to head and neck, and of *Ang. 2* to heart, and *Ang. 3* ointment to head and neck.

3. If resulting from passive congestion, in cases of anæmia, asthma, valvular heart disease, sluggish liver, &c., the treatment should be directed to the cure of these diseases, and compress of *Ang. 3* be applied to the head and neck.

4. In rheumatic headache, *Scrof. 1*, litre dil. alt. *Ang. 3*, second dil. Compress of *Canc. 5*, *White*, *Blue*, or *Green* El. Apply *Blue* or *Yellow* El. to 17, 18, and *Canc. 5*, *Scrof.*, *Ang. 3*, or *Scrof. 5* ointment to head.

5. In headache resulting from uterine derangement, give *Canc. 1*, second dil. Apply *Canc. 5* ointment to head and take *Canc. 1* or *5* baths, especially sitz-baths. *White* El. to centre of cranium.

6. In headache resulting from mental or physical overwork, give *Scrof. 1*, litre dil. (or in the cases of women, *Canc. 1*, litre dil.) and apply ointment and compress of *Scrof.* alt. *Canc. 5*. Baths of *White* or *Green* El. *White* El. to centre of cranium.

7. In cases of chronic heaadche give *Scrof. 1*, second dil. Apply compress *Canc. 5*. Ointment of *Scrof.* and *Canc. 5* to 6 and forehead. Apply *Red* alt. *Yellow* or *White* El. or *Canc. 5* to 5, 6, 17, 18. Baths *Canc. 5*.

8. In periodical headaches (Hemicrania): *Feb. 1*, third dil. Apply *Feb. 2* alt. *Canc. 5* to 24.

In all cases of headache one or other of the electricities is useful and should be applied to 17, 18, 1, 2, 3, 6, 23, and behind the ears, and to the temples. Also to soles of feet. *White or Green* El. is most generally useful. *Blue* El. is valuable in congestive headaches, and in some cases *Red* alt. *Yellow* El. may be used.

Heart: The central organ in the body is liable to numerous affections. Most of these are of so serious a nature that it is advisable to seek the guidance of a competent medical man in all cases where their existence is suspected. The following are some of the principal forms of organic heart disease.

(i.) *Acute inflammations.* (*a*) Of the pericardium (Pericarditis). This occurs chiefly in the course of rheumatic fever or Bright's disease. An attack is accompanied by tenderness, palpitation, and more or less intense pain. The heart's impulse gives evidence of excitement. Fluid accumulates in the pericardium, which produces bulging, difficulty of breathing, and sometimes a dry spasmodic cough.

(*b*.) *Acute inflammation* of the endocardium (Endocarditis) resulting from the presence of a morbid poison in the blood. The heart's action is excited. There are endocardial murmurs and there sometimes is mitral regurgitation.

(*c.*) *Acute inflammation* of the heart substance itself (Myocarditis).

(ii.) *Chronic inflammations.* These include chronic pericarditis, endocartitis and myocarditis and give rise to organic mischief in the valves or their appendages, or in the cardiac orifices, and so permit part of the blood which has been driven through the valves to flow back again or obstruct the flow of the stream through the valves. Any of the valves may thus be affected. The mitral valve may be so injured that *mitral regurgitation* follows, the supply of blood to the arterial system is decreased and the pulse becomes small, weak, and unequal. The left auricle becomes dilated aud hypertrophied, and other evils supervene. If the orifice is constricted there is *mitral obstruction.* In this case the pulse is regular and the left ventricle tends to become atrophied. *Aortic obstruction* induces anæmia, tendency to syncope, and want of vigour, coldness of extremities, and hypertrophy of the left ventricle. *Aortic regurgitation* is attended by a jerky pulse, producing a sensation as if balls of blood were shot under the finger, and gives rise to serious hypertrophy and dilatation of the left ventricle. *Tricuspid regurgitation* leads to overloading of the veins, dropsy, hypertrophy of the right auricle and ventricle. Tricuspid obstruction and diseases of the pulmonary valves are very rare. The walls of the heart may be enlarged and the cavities may be dilated. Pure hypertrophy may not give rise to any symptoms. If, however, it is excessive, the arteries become distended, and tend to degenerate, and there is bulging over the heart. Hypertrophy of the left ventricle generally gives rise to throbbing of the arteries.

If it is insufficient then there is palpitation and difficulty of breathing, with occasional irregularity of the heart's action. When there is much dilatation there are symptoms of venous congestion, pain over the cardiac region, and dyspnœa. Another disease to which the heart walls are liable is fatty degeneration, a condition which often results from hypertrophy or dilatation of the heart. In this affection the heart beats are greatly reduced, the patient feels weak and depressed, his breathing becomes disturbed, he is liable to attacks of giddiness, and is subject to involuntary sighing.

In all chronic heart cases patients should avoid hurry, straining, strong emotions, excesses, and should be careful to restrict their diet to such articles as they can easily digest. They should be warmly clad.

A great many persons believe that their hearts are diseased who are suffering only from disturbed action of the heart in consequence of flatulent dyspepsia, hæmic or blood diseases, anæmia, gout, chlorosis, reflex irritation, &c. Palpitation may be caused by acute or chronic diseases of the heart or pericardium, mechanical interference with the heart's action (as by tight corsets), excess or deficiency of blood, morbid states of the blood, hypochondriasis, gout, and nervous excitement. A fit of palpitation may be accompanied by increased frequency and force of the heart's beat, sensation as if the heart were jumping up into the throat, faintness, cold extremities, and even a feeling as if death were approaching.

In functional disorders of the heart *Feb. 1*, second or litre dil., will be found useful, with *Feb. 2* ointment to 24.

In organic diseases of the heart treatment should be

begun with *Ang. 3* ointment lightly applied to the cardiac region, and in cases where there is no rheumatic tendency, compresses of *Ang. 3* or *Ang. 2* (2 globules to quarter of a pint of water) may be worn. The tips of three fingers or the palm of the right hand may be moistened with 5 drops of ***Blue*** El. and passed gently over the heart. After a day or two a dry globule of *Ang. 3* may be given every 2 or 3 hours. Subsequently *Ang. 3*, second or third dil. may be taken alone, or in alternation with *Canc. 1*, second dil. When there are rheumatic complications *Scrof. 1* or *2*, second or third dil. should be alternated with *Ang. 3*, third dil. In some instances tepid baths of *Ang. 3* or *Canc. 5* may be taken. To relieve palpitation rub a little *Blue* El. lightly on the cardiac region.

Heartburn (Cardialgia): a burning sensation which extends upwards from the epigastrium to the throat or sometimes over the abdomen. It occurs in cases of dilatation of the stomach, chronic catarrhal gastritis, and often during pregnancy. Fatty and starchy foods should be avoided. *Scrof.* or *Canc. 5*, litre dil., alt. *Ang.*, second dil. Applications of *White* El. to 6, and of *Yellow* El. to 17, 18. Compress of *White* or ***Blue*** El. to 6, or *Canc. 5* ointment over the stomach.

Helminthiasis: See Worms.

Hemicrania, better known as sick headache, or megrim: an obscure neuralgic affection believed by some to be due to nerve storms to which ladies are especially liable. The attacks are periodic and are generally ushered in by sensations of uneasiness, irritability, distaste for food, &c. The pain is usually limited to one side, and is ordinarily of a throbbing character. After a while nausea and vomiting set in. *Feb. 1*, second dil. alt. *Scrof. 1*, second dil. Application of *Canc. 5* ointment over the head and neck, and of *White* El. to 16, 17, 18. Light compress of *White* El. to cranium, or compress of *Green* El. If there are symptoms of congestion use *Ang. 1*, second dil., instead of *Scrof.*, and *Ang. 3* ointment instead of *Canc. 5*. *Feb. 2* ointment to 24 and *Ang. 3* to heart. Applications of *Blue* El. to 16, 17, 18. Baths of *Ang. 3*. If supposed to originate in uterine disorders or in leucorrhœa, *Canc. 1*, second dil.; 1 globule *Canc. 5* hourly. Compress of *Green* El. Baths of *Canc. 5*. Application of *White* El. to 17, 18, and soles of feet. If occurring at menstrual periods, 2 globules *Scrof.* night and morning, with *Canc.*, third dil., alt. *Scrof. 1*, second dil.

Hemiplegia: Paralysis of motion or of motion and sensation of one side of the body: See Paralysis.

Hepatic Abscess: Acute inflammation of the liver tissue ending in suppuration, resulting from injury to the liver, irritation, intense heat, &c. It is accompanied by dull aching, or throbbing pain, and produces local bulging. When suppuration sets in, there are rigors, feverishness, and prostration. *Feb. 1*, second dil., alt. *Scrof. 1*, or, in sanguine patients, *Ang. 3* or *2*, litre dil., 1 globule *Canc.* hourly, *Feb. 2* and *Canc. 5* compress and ointment to 24.

Hernia: See Rupture.

Herpes: an acute skin disease of which there are several varieties, one of which, affecting the trunk, is popularly known as shingles. It usually begins with a pricking burning pain, and the appearance of red points. Their contents become turbid and they themselves then dry up. In about ten days small brownish scabs fall off.

In some cases the disease is periodic. *Scrof. 1*, second or third dil., with baths of *Scrof. 1* alt. *Scrof.* 5.

Hooping (or Whooping) **Cough**: an infectious disease, to which children under eight years of age are specially liable, and which is highly fatal to young infants. The infectious particles may be carried in visitors' clothes from house to house. The invasion stage lasts a week. There are catarrh, loss of appetite, bronchial *râles*, and feverish symptoms. The whoop usually begins on the tenth day, but may be delayed much longer. When the cough is coming the child's face reddens. Then follows a series of short efforts, a shrill whistling sound is heard as the breath is drawn in, a boisterous cough follows, two shorter fits of coughing follows, and at last a sour whitish viscid mucus is expelled. The disease usually lasts several weeks. *Ang. 1*, third dil. alt *Pet. 3*, third dil. alt. *Canc. 1*, third dil., or *Canc. 5*, third dil. Some practitioners advise mixing the remedies together in a glass of milk from which the child takes frequent sips during the day. Baths of *Canc. 5*. *White* El., *Ang. 3* ointment to heart. *Blue* El. to 5, 13, 18.

Hydatid Tumour: a tumour of the liver, originating in the development of the embryos of a particular form of tape worm. The tumour is usually spherical in shape, and occupies the right lobe of the liver. Sometimes it grows to an enormous size and produces atrophy of the surrounding tissue. It produces an increase of the size of the liver, a change in its form, and a sense of local fulness or tension. *Feb. 1*, second dil., alt. *Ang. 3* or *2*, litre dil.; 1 globule *Canc. 1* hourly. *Feb. 2* compress, and ointment to 24. *White* El. compress over loins. *Ang. 3* ointment to heart. Baths *Ang. 3* alt. *Feb. 2.* Applications *Red* alt. *Yellow* El. to 5, 18, and also to liver and spleen.

Hydrocele: a collection of fluid in connection with the testicle or spermatic cord. *Scrof. 1* or *5* alt. *Canc. 2* or *4.* Frictions of *White* El. Baths of *Canc. 5*, *Scrof. 1*, or *Ang. 3.* Compress of *Canc. 5. Red* El. to 20, 22. *White* El. to cranium. Enemata with 20 globules of *Canc. 5.* Sitz-baths of *Lin.*

Hydrocephalus: The acute form of this disease is due to irritation, caused by the presence of tubercles in the membranes of the brain. It most commonly attacks children from 2 to 10 years of age. Its victims show signs of ill-health for some time before the invasion symptoms appear. They are specially liable to drowsiness, sudden screaming and starting, and headache. Sometimes the disease developes very slowly. At other times the invasion is very sudden. There is much frontal headache and intolerance of light and sound. The gait is unsteady, the pupils contract and dilate, sleep is disturbed. There is some feverishness. As the disease advances, the eyeballs and pupils oscillate, the patient assumes an aged look and sighs or moans rather than breathes. Other and more serious symptoms manifest themselves as the disease advances to its final stage. *Scrof. 1*, second dil. or *Canc. 1*, third dil. alt. *Ang. 3*, second or third dil. *Canc. 5* or *Lin.* ointment to head. *Feb. 2* ointment to 24. *Blue* or *White* El. to centre of cranium. *Yellow* El. to 5, 17, 18, and nerves of head.

The chronic form of this disease, is popularly known as "water on the brain." The heads of children who suffer from this complaint are much enlarged, and the lower part of the face seems small. The mental faculties, if they develope at all, gradually fail. Sleep is disturbed, co-ordinating power is lost, and the body wastes. *Scrof.* second dil. alt. *Ang. 2*, third dil. Compress of *Canc. 5*. Application of *Blue* El. to centre of cranium, and chief nerve centres.

Hydrophobia : an acute disease caused by inoculation with the poison of a rabid dog, cat, fox or wolf. At first there are malaise, depression, and a difficulty in swallowing liquids. Spasm in the throat follows, which becomes so intense and so easily excited that the patient cannot bear the sight or even the sound of water. The saliva is ejected with a barking noise. The patient should at once have a vapour bath, and may try *Scrof. 1* or *5*, litre dil. Applications of *Red* El. alt. *Yellow* El. to 18, 17, 5, 6.

Hydrops : See Dropsy.

Hyperæmia. Excess of blood. It may be general or local. It may be active or arterial on the one hand, or passive or venous on the other. *Ang. 1* or *3*, second or third dil. Compress of *Ang. 3* over the heart. The lotion for the compresses should be made by dissolving 2 globules of *Ang. 1* or *2* in from a teaspoonful to a tablespoonful of water.

Hypochondriasis : The subjects of this affection imagine that they suffer from some organic disease and are very fond of taking medicine and of consulting doctors. *Canc. 1*, second or third dil. alt. *Feb. 1*, second dil.; 2 drops of *Blue* El. twice a day. Baths of *Canc. 5*. *Feb. 2* ointment to 24. In some cases *Scrof. 1* or *Ang.* may be substituted for *Feb.*

Hysteria: a nervous disorder which may result from defective nutrition of the nervous system. Ladies, especially young ladies, suffer from this much more frequently than men. Its victims, in most cases, are subject to hysterical fits which are preceded by sighing and sobbing, and are accompanied by noisy and irregular breathing, spasmodic movements, &c. These patients are also subject to great fluctuation of spirits. As a rule they devote a great deal of attention to themselves, and are never so happy as when they can induce others to turn their thoughts in the same direction. They are often impatient and irritable. They are extremely sensitive, and are subject to a peculiar sensation (clavus hystericus) which seems as if a nail were in their skull. Cramp and even paralysis sometimes occur. Loss of voice is a frequent symptom. Hysterical patients are liable to imagine that they suffer from spinal disease, tumours, &c. Patients of lymphatic temperament should take a few teaspoonfuls daily of *Canc. 1*, second dil. or *Canc. 2*, second dil. alt. *Scrof.*, second or third dil., or *Scrof. 2*, with 2 drops of *Yellow* El. night and morning. Patients of mixed and sanguine temperaments require 2 globules of *Scrof. 2* dry on the tongue in the morning. A few teaspoonfuls of *Canc.*, third dil. alt. *Ang. 2*, third dil., and 2 drops of *Yellow* or *Blue* El. in the evening, with *Ang. 2* ointment on the heart. In cases which do not yield to this treatment, *Ver.* or *Ven.* should be tried. In all cases baths of *Scrof.* or *Ang 3* or *2*, alt. *Canc. 5* or of *Lin.* may be taken. Special care must be taken to avoid taking more than from 4 to 8 teaspoonfuls of each remedy per diem. A lotion of *White* El. is useful in the treatment of clavus hystericus. The application of *Blue* El. to 6 has cut short hysterical crises.

Icthyosis : a skin disease characterised by the breaking-up of the cuticle into sections which resemble the scales of a fish. For treatment see Eczema.

Icterus : See Jaundice.

Idiocy : Feeble-mindedness in early childhood. Its subjects are generally small physically as well as intellectually. Their senses are defective and their power of co-ordination is small. Some are born idiots. Others become such at the time of the first or second dentition or at the period of puberty. An accident or an attack of disease of the bones of the ear or rickets may lead to it. *Canc 1*, third dil. Compress of *White* El. to 20. *Red* alt. *Yellow* to 5, 17, 18, and nerves of head. *White* El. to both sides of spine.

Ileus : See Intestinal Obstruction.

Impetigo : An eruption of small pustular vesicles which are but slightly inflamed. In some cases they are as small as a pin's head. In others they are a quarter of an inch in diameter. After a few days the secretion forms a brownish-yellow crust. Sometimes, especially when associated with eczema, it forms a large crust. It is then known as milk crust. *Scrof. 1*, second or third dil. or alt. with *Ang. 3*, third dil. Baths of *Scrof. 1* alt. *Canc. 5*. *Scrof. 5* ointment.

Impetigo Contagiosa : A contagious variety of the above disease, which is sometimes epidemic and occasionally accompanied by symptoms of feverishness. Same treatment.

Impotence : a condition which may result from sexual excess, diseases of the brain or spinal cord, kidney diseases, varicocele, &c. 5 globules *Canc. 4* or *5* night and morning; *Scrof. 1* litre dil., *Lin.* second dil. Application *Red* alt. *Yellow* El. to 6, 17, 18, 20. Baths of *Red* and *Blue* El.

Incontinence of Urine: See Urine.

Indigestion: See Dyspepsia.

Infantile Paralysis: See Paralysis.

Inflammation: For most inflammations *Scrof. 1* or *Canc. 1*, if suppuration has set in, in the second or third dil., with compresses of the same remedies will prove efficacious. When the inflammation is accompanied by fever, *Feb.* must be added. It may be noted that *Canc. 1* in the first dil. promotes suppuration, and that in the third dil. it diminishes it.

Inflammation of Lungs: See Lungs.

Influenza: an epidemic catarrhal fever, which, in its simple form, suddenly attacks the patient, produces a sense of cold in the back, followed by flushes of heat, sore throat, a sense of tightness in the chest, distressing headache, prostration of strength and sometimes pains in the limbs. The tongue is moist and covered with a creamy fur. At first there is but little expectoration, but afterwards a great deal of opaque mucus is coughed up. In the graver form of the disease the pains in the limbs are very marked, and the bronchial tubes and lungs are usually more seriously affected. If acute capillary bronchitis sets in the rate of the pulse rises to 110 or 116. Frontal headache is much complained of, and there is considerable pain in the back and limbs. The pulse beats 120 to 140 times per minute. The respirations per minute rise to 30 and upwards. The lips become purplish. Should the disease not be checked dyspnœa becomes severe. The cheeks become livid and the eyes stand out. An anxious expression is worn by the patient. If the disease is complicated with gastro-intestinal affections and rheumatism there is much bilious vomiting, and the pains in the head, back, and limbs are very severe. The pulse is feeble and intermittent. The perspiration has an acid smell. Profuse perspiration follows and the patient becomes very prostrate. To prevent the disease take 5 globs. *Scrof.* night and morning, and 5 globs. *Scrof. Giap.* at meals. Gargles of *Scrof.* To cure it go to bed and take a massive dose of *Feb. 1* (5 to 10 globs. in a wineglassful of water) at a single dose, or of *Scrof. Giap.*, and then *Feb. 1*, second dil. or third dil. if the fever is very high. This may be alternated with *Scrof. Giap.* and *Canc. 5. Feb. 2* compress and ointment to 24. *Canc. 5* ointment to 24 and back. Blanket-pack or wet-pack is useful. To relieve pains of head and back use compress of *White* El. To subdue cough and check inflammation take *Ang. 3*, second dil. alt. *Pet. 2*, second dil. alt. *Canc. 1*, second dil.; 2 drops of *White* El. hourly till fever subsides. Gargles of *Blue* El. Be careful to avoid chills during convalescence.

Insanity : a mental disorder resulting from injury to or defect in the development of some part of the organs of the intellect, from insufficient nerve force, from too great demands being made upon the supply or from an unstable condition of the brain centres. At first, there is sleeplessness, followed, it may be, only by dulness or excitability, or also by gloominess or violence. Delusions or childishness may supervene.

In cases where there is excitability, *Ang. 3*, should be

given alt. *Canc. 1*, second or third dil. Whenever there is gloominess, give *Scrof. 1*, second or third dil., alternated, in the case of women, with *Canc. 1*, second dil. Baths of *Canc. 5*. In some cases *White* El. may be applied to 17, 18, and in melancholia to back of neck.

Much may be done by means of music and colour. Certain kinds of these have a singularly beneficial effect upon the insane. Violet colour and soft music will calm excited nerves, just as red colour and rapid music will increase excitability.

Insomnia (Sleeplessness: 3 to 5 globs. *Scrof. 1* or *2* or, in some cases, 1 glob. *Ang. 2* dry on tongue at night. Applications of *Red* El. to 5, 17, 18. If the insomnia arises from a febrile state of blood, take *Feb. 1*, second dil., every evening.

Intercostal Neuralgia: See Neuralgia.

Intermittent Fever: See Fever.

Intertrigo: Inflammation of the skin in the hollows or folds of joints caused by local friction, heat or moisture. Care should be taken to remove the cause. Treat like Eczema.

Intestinal Obstruction: Hindrance of the passage of fœcal matter through the intestines, caused by malformation, strangulation, gall-stones, constriction, compression, the passage of one portion of the intestine into the immediately adjoining part, or the accumulation of fœcal masses. The symptoms include pain, distress, vomiting, constipation, and distension of the abdomen about the seat of obstruction. The patient's face becomes livid, and the lips pale or purplish. His temperature usually sinks below normal but rises if peritonitis sets in. He is tormented with thirst, and in many cases suffers from distressing hiccough.

The treatment differs according to the cause. Ordinarily, however, 5 globs. *Scrof. 1* may be given dry every hour, and *Scrof. 1* or *Canc. 1* in second or third dil. every 10 minutes. A more or less copious enema of gruel or olive oil medicated with 15 globs. of *Canc. 5* to the half-pint. Or a glycerine enema by means of a special syringe. Massage and hot fomentations medicated with *Canc. 5* are serviceable.

Intestines: The diagnosis of intestinal diseases is difficult.

Cancer in the intestines: See Cancer.

Catarrh of the intestines should be treated like inflammation of the intestines.

Hæmorrhage from the intestines should be treated according to its cause, whether this be extreme congestion or hyperæmia, injuries of the bowels, ulceration, piles, vicarious menstruation, &c.

Inflammation of the intestines: See Enteritis.

Paralysis of the intestines: See Paralysis.

Spasm of the intestines: See Spasms.

Tubercular disease of the intestine: See Tuberculosis.

Ulceration of the intestines: This may result from any form of intestinal inflammation, and gives rise to the presence of blood in the stools.

Itch: *Scrof.*, second dil., or *Canc. 1*, second dil. alt. *Ang. 2*. *Red* alt. *Yellow* El. to 5, 18, 17. Baths of *Canc. 5*, *White* El. and *Ang. 3*. Ointment of *Canc. 5* or *Feb. 2* to 24.

Jaundice: a yellowness of the integuments conjunctivæ, tissues, and secretions, arising from their impregnation with bile pigment. It is a symptom of many varied diseases rather than a disease in itself, and the treatment should be directed to the fundamental malady. In simple cases the chief remedies are *Feb. 1*, first or litre dil. *Feb. 2* ointment or compress to 24. Compress of *Canc. 5* over liver.

Joints: Affection of the joints include the following:

Synovitis: The membrane which lines the joints and which supplies them with the fluid by means of which they are lubricated is liable both to acute and chronic inflammations. The former very frequently result from injury. There are three varieties of it: the serous, the sero-fibrinous and the purulent. The first is the commonest. The membrane becomes thickened. The tissue beneath it becomes œdematous. The pressure of the effused fluid causes bulging. There are symptoms of feverishness. In the chronic variety which may follow the acute form or result from certain constitutional conditions, there is a uniform semi-elastic swelling, with smooth and whitish skin (white swelling). *Scrof. 1*, first or litre dil. Compress, ointment and baths of *Scrof. 1* alt. *Scrof. 5*, with 5 globs. *Scrof. 1* at meals. When suppuration commences alt. *Canc. 1* with *Scrof. 1*, and use baths and compresses of *Canc. 5*.

Gouty inflammation of the joints sometimes results from the deposit of urate of soda in the tissue which surrounds the synovial membrane. For treatment see Gout.

Nervous affections of joints or hysterical affections simulating joint disease sometimes occur. Treatment as in Hysteria.

Scrofulous inflammation should be treated like Scrofula.

Syphilitic diseases of: Treat like Syphilis.

Kidneys, Diseases of: These important organs are liable to a great variety of diseases of which a few only can be mentioned here. It may be observed, however, that *Feb. 1*, *Scrof. 6* and *Canc. 6* are generally useful in the treatment of kidney diseases.

Bright's Disease: See Albuminuria.

Congestion of the Kidney: When this occurs in its active form there is albumin in the urine. In its passive form the urine is scanty and highly coloured. *Ang.* alt. *Feb. 1*.

Inflammation of the pelvis of the kidney (Pyelitis): There are three forms of this: the acute, the chronic, and the calculous. The first produces a sensation of uneasiness or pain in the loins; the second causes also constitutional disturbance; the third produces more pain than either of the others. *Feb. 1* alt. *Scrof.* *Lin.* ointment, compress and bath.

King's Evil: See Scrofula.

Laryngitis: Inflammation of the mucous membrane of the larynx. There is a sense of constriction, or hissing breathing, a croaking voice and a rapid pulse. The acute stridulous form resembles croup. It must be remembered that many laryngeal affections are secondary to lung troubles. At first, if there is feverishness, use *Feb. 1*, second or third dil., with *Feb. 2* ointment to 24. *Domfin*, second dil. alt. *Scrof. 1*, second dil. Apply *Red* alt. *Yellow* El. to 18, 17. Gargles of *Red*, *White* El., *Domfin*, *Canc. 5*, or *Scrof.* At first ointment of *Ang. 3* alt. *Domfin*. Then *Domfin* ointment alt. *Canc. 5* ointment. Afterwards *Canc. 5* and *Scrof. 5* ointment.

Chronic laryingitis produces hoarseness, and loss of voice, a hacking cough, and a sense of dryness and pain in the throat. *Scrof.*, second or third dil. alt. *Domfin*, second dil. If obstinate *Pet. 1* alt. *Canc. 5* ointment. *Red* El. gargles. Compress of *Domfin.*

Spasmodic laryngitis exhibits the same symptoms as as chronic laryngitis, with the addition of œdema and ulceration : *Canc. 5*, second dil. alt. *Domfin*, second dil. 1 glob. *Pet. 1* dry hourly. *Domfin* compress and gargles, and gargles of *Canc. 1* alt. *Canc. 5.*

Syphilitic laryngitis : For treatment see Syphilis. *Pet. 1* alt. *Ang. 3* alt. *Canc. 5*, and 1 dry glob. of *Ven.* every 1 or 2 hours. Gargles of *Ven.* alt. *Canc. 5* and *Green* El. Care must be taken not to swallow any of the *Green* El. To make gargles add 3 drops El. and 3 globs. to 1 ounce of water and a quarter of an ounce of glycerine.

Leprosy : a disease which chiefly affects the skin and the nervous system. At first, there are dull copper-coloured circular spots or irregularly shaped blotches indicative of local congestions. Then subside and leave a pigmentary stain. The tubercles then assume other forms. The skin becomes thickened. Its sensibility decreases. The hair falls. For two weeks give *Scrof. 1* or *2*, third dil. alt. *Canc. 5*, third dil., 10 drops every five minutes. When the circulatory system is affected add *Ang. 1*, third dil. Baths of *Lin.* alt. *Ven.* alt. *Canc. 5.*

Leucorrhœa (The Whites) : a white discharge from the female genitals, which may originate in the vulva, the vagina, the cervix uteri, or the uterus itself. Take 1 glob. *Canc. 5* hourly ; *Scrof. 1*, litre or second dil. alt. *Canc.*, second dil., or, in sanguine temperaments, *Ang. 3*, litre or second dil. alt. *Canc.*, second dil. *Lin.* ointment alt. *Scrof. 5* ointment relieves the weary pains in the back. Baths of *Scrof. 5.* Injections of *Canc. 5.* In obstinate cases *Ang. 2* litre dil. alt. *Canc. 5*, litre dil. If this does not effect a cure give *Ven.* or *Verm.* according as the presence of a syphilitic taint or of worms is suspected.

Legs, Swelling of: *Ang. 1* or *2*, second dil. alt. *Canc. 2*, second dil. Ointment or lotion of *Ang. 3.* Application of *Blue* El. to 18, 17. Baths of *Ang. 3. Feb. 2* ointment to 24.

Cancer of: See Cancer.

Cirrhosis of: A disease leading to contraction and wasting of the liver. The surface of this organ becomes pale and is covered with a series of granules resembling hob-nails. In most cases it is caused by abuse of alcohol. But it may originate otherwise. *Feb. 1*, second or third dil. *Feb. 2* ointment to 24. Should the veins of the abdomen be enlarged give 5 globules *Canc. 5* morning and evening, and *Ang. 2*, second dil. alt. *Feb. 1*, second or third dil., and rub *Feb. 2* ointment alt *Canc. 5* ointment over 24. In obstinate cases add 1 glob. *Canc. 5* hourly, or a few teaspoonfuls of *Canc. 1* second or third dil. per diem.

Congestion of: This produces a sense of discomfort and weight in the region of the liver. Besides this there often may be observed slight jaundice, pain in the right shoulder, and impaired appetite. It may be caused by the abuse of rich food or alcoholic beverages, excessive heat or sudden chills, &c. *Feb. 1*, second dil. alt. *Ang. 2*, litre dil. *Feb. 2* ointment and compress to 24. *Ang. 3* ointment to heart. *Red* alt. *Yellow* or *White* El. to liver region. Baths of *Ang. 3* alt. *Feb. 2.*

Inflammation of (Hepatitis) acute : An extremely fatal disease, probably commencing with the presence of an excess of blood in the organ, followed by the effusion of lymph, degeneration of the liver cells, and the formation of abscesses. The patient experiences rigors and becomes feverish. He feels dull aching pain and tenderness over the liver region. There is derangement of the alimentary canal. *Feb. 1*, second dil. alt. *Scrof.* 1, second dil. Compress of *Canc. 5*. Ointment of *Feb. 2* to 24. Apply *Red* alt. *Yellow* El. to 5, 18, 17, and *White* El. to liver region. Should an abscess form substitute *Canc. 1* for *Scrof. 1*, and alt. *Canc. 5* ointment with *Feb. 2.*

Ulceration of : See Ulcers.

Lockjaw (Trismus) : Persistent spasm or rigidity of the muscles behind the neck and subsequently of othe voluntary muscles, often accompanied by backward curvature of the body. There is an agonising sense of constriction in the stomach. Fits of spasm occur, attended by cessation of breath, and excessive perspiration. The pupils are dilated. 10 globs. *Scrof.* ; *Scrof. 1*, first or second dil. Application of *Yellow* El. or of *Yellow* alt. *Red* El. to masseter muscle and to 18, 17. Compress of *Canc. 5* alt. *White* El. Baths of *Canc. 5* alt. *Lin.* Ointment of *Canc. 5* alt. *Scrof.* When contraction becomes general a mixture of *Scrof. 1*, first dil., *Ver.* 1, first dil. and 10 to 20 drops of *Yellow* El. may be given in small doses.

Locomotor ataxy : Degeneration of the posterior column of the spinal cord, leading to loss of power of co-ordination in the muscles of the legs. It may be caused by exposure or excesses. It is preceded by sensory and sexual disturbance, neuralgic pains, &c. Treat like Paralysis.

Lumbago: Muscular rheumatism in the lumbar region. Treat like rheumatism, with *Scrof.* in litre or second dil., adding *Feb. 1*, second or third dil., if there is feverishness and *Ver.* Compress of *Canc. 5*, *Scrof. 5* or *White* El. Applications of *Red* alt. *Yellow* El. to 5, 18, 17, and sides of spine. Rub *Red* El. well over kidneys and sacral region. Ointment of *Scrof. 5* alt. *Canc. 5* or *Lin.* and baths of same.

Lungs: See Cough, Consumption, Phthisis.

Catarrhal inflammation of the lungs (Broncho-pneumonia): In this variety of the disease the inflammation of the lung tissue is accompanied by inflammation of the mucous membrane of the bronchi. Its symptoms resemble those of Bronchitis, capillary (which see). There are frequent cough, rapid shallow breathing, or high temperature (104°), quick pulse.

Cirrhosis of: Chronic pneumonia or intertial pneumonia. *Scrof. 1*, second dil. alt. *Pet. 2*, second dil. alt. *Ang. 3*, second dil. *Canc. 5* ointment.

Emphysema of: Distension of the air-sacs or the presence of air in the interlobular tissue. The size of the upper part of the chest increases. Inspiration causes but little increase in size and is short, quick, and followed by a long expiration. There is increased resonance over the chest. *Scrof. 1*, litre dil.

Gangrene of: Death of a part of the lung-tissue. In the diffused kind the whole of one lobe is affected; in the circumscribed kind a part only of one lobe is gangrened. See Gangrene.

Hepatization: *Canc. 2* and *Canc. 5* ointment and inhalation.

Inflammation of (Pneumonia) Acute: Inflammation of the lung tissue. At first there is engorgement. The lung increases in size and becomes hardened and of a reddish brown colour. It afterwards becomes grey. As a rule only one lung is affected. The invasion of the disease is indicated by a marked rigor. High fever, insomnia, frequent respiration but a comparatively slow pulse, pain in the side, loss of appetite, diminished secretion of urine are characteristic symptoms. In the congestive stage of the disease there may be heard in the chest a peculiar sound which has been compared to the sound produced by rubbing the hair between the fingers close to the ear. Attack the initiatory fever with *Feb. 1*, second or third dil. with *Feb. 2* compress and ointment. When the inflammation begins, 1 glob. *Canc.* hourly. *Scrof.* litre or second dil. alt. *Pet. 1* or *2*, second dil. alt. *Ang. 3*, second or third dil., teaspoonfuls every 5 minutes. Weak applications of *Red* El. to 5, 6 and 18. 1 glob. *Pet. 1* dry hourly, if there is much coughing. *Pet. 1* ointment or oil to chest. *Canc. 5* ointment or oil to back. *Feb. 2* ointment to 24.

Inflammation of (chronic): See Lungs, cirrhosis of.

Tuberculosis: *Pet. 1* or *Pet. 2*, second dil. alt. *Canc.*, second dil. alt. *Ang. 3*. 5 globs. *Scrof. Giap.* at meals. *Pet. 3* alt. *Canc. 5* ointment to chest.

Lupus: A growth of tuberculous tissue on the face or other part of the body, which appears sometimes in an non-ulcerative form. At first there are some small reddish blotches or nodules. In the non-ulcerative form thin whitish scales appear, which fall off. The ulcerative form attacks deep-seated tissues as well as the skin, and sometimes destroys the whole of a patient's nose. Begin with *Scrof. 5*, first or second dil., with compress of *Scrof. 1* alt. *Scrof. 5*. Afterwards *Canc. 1* or *4*, second or third dil. alt. *Ang. 2*, third dil., if there is any hæmorrhage. If syphilitic complications are suspected add *Ven.*, second dil. Compress and daily baths of *Canc. 5* or *1*, alt. *Lin.* Finish treatment with *Scrof. 5*, litre dil. and compress of *Scrof 5* alt. *Green* El.

Malaria : See Fevers.

Mania : See Insanity.

Marasmus, General wasting : *Scrof. 1*, litre or second dil. *Red* alt. *Yellow* El. to 5, 18, 17. *White* El. to head. *Canc. 5* ointment to head. Dr. Kennedy advises frictions of mutton suet melted with *Canc. 5*. Take finely minced mutton suet dissolved in warm milk every 2 hours.

Masturbation (Self-abuse) : A very common vice, against which parents should carefully warn their children, as these are taught the practice at school, and form the fatal habit without any idea of its criminality or physical hurtfulness. The effects include perversion of the nervous functions, loss of memory, despondency, anæmia, disturbance of the heart's action, discharge of prostatic secretions. Treatment must include moral suasion, and be directed to the improvement of the general health. *Scrof. 1* dil., *Lin.* ointment to 20.

Measles : A fever originating from infection by means of bacteria which may be carried in clothing, &c. The early symptoms include sneezing, watery eyes, cough, and sometimes vomiting. The temperature gradually rises. Pinkish-red points soon appear on the face and feel like shot beneath the skin. They form crescentic blotches.

The patient's eye is tender and watery. The lymphatic glands of the neck are enlarged. The tongue is furred. The rash continues to spread for two or three days and remains three days or more. As the rash declines small bran-like scales of cuticle fall off. Bronchial complications, or pneumonia, are among the sequelæ which are most to be dreaded. In the early treatment of the disease the wet pack is very valuable. But great care must be taken to do the packing in the right way. Otherwise grave evils may follow. The patient should be kept in bed in a warm room. During convalescence care must be taken to avoid exposure to draught. To reduce the fever, give an occasional teaspoonful of *Feb. 1*, second or third dil. Compress of *Feb. 2* to 24. No waterproof material is is to be used. If the pulse is very high and the symptoms marked, a large compress of *Canc. 5* should be applied to the head and changed as soon as dry. While the fever is very high give 5 globs. *Scrof.* dry every half-hour; then the litre dil. of *Scrof. 1* in teaspoonfuls every five minutes. Not much *Feb. 1* should be used. Apply *Red* El. to 17, 1, temples, and soles of feet. After the fever is reduced give *Scrof. 1*, first dil., to bring out the eruption. Should the eruption suddenly re-enter put, if necessary, 2 globs. of *Scrof. 1* in the glass, or, if this fails to bring it back, a massive dose (20 globs.) of *Scrof. 1* every hour until it come out again. Bronchial and other complications must be treated as they arise. A light diet is needed so long as fever exists.

Megrim: See Migraine.

Melæna: Hæmorrhage from the intestines which may originate in the stomach, or may result from injury, vitiations of the blood, various organic diseases especially piles, tumours, aneurisms, ulcers, &c. Treatment varies with the cause. A few teaspoonfuls of *Ang. 3* in third dil. may be given daily. Sitz baths of *Ang. 3* are of use in most cases. *Ang. 3*, second dil. or *Ang. 2*, second dil., sometimes alt. with *Canc. 1*, second dil. Compress of *Blue* and *Ang. 3* to 27. *Blue* El. to 5, 18, 17. Sitz baths of *Ang. 3*. 2 or 3 drops of *Blue* El. on sugar 2 or 3 times daily.

Melancholia : A form of insanity characterised by great mental depression. Its victims usually suffer from obstinate constipation, loss of flesh and insomnia. *Scrof. 1*, third dil. If arising from uterine disorders *Canc. 2*, third dil., and *Red* El. to 20, 22, 5, 18.

Menieère's Disease (Auditory Vertigo) : Vertigo caused by disturbance of the functions of that part of the ear which is known as the labyrinth (See Ear : diseases of.) The patient hears loud noises in the ear, experiences feelings of giddiness and nausea. The first attack leaves more or less deafness behind it. Some forms of this disease are curable with *Scrof. 5* third dil. and *White* El. Others result from irremediable affections of the labyrinth.

Meningeal Hæmorrhage : Hæmorrhage into the meninges, generally resulting from strain, injury, or the rupture of an aneurism, or of an artery. The more severe attacks cause apoplectic symptoms. *Ang. 3*, third dil. 2 drops of *Blue* El. every 2 hours.

Meningitis : Inflammation of the membranes of the brain, resulting from injury, bone disease, exposure to direct solar rays, &c.

Acute : Preceded by vertigo, or irritability. The

invasion is attended by rigor, feverishness, headache, and vomiting. Then follows a stage of excitement, during which there are intense headache, darting pains, delirium and fever. Afterwards, in fatal cases, come spasms, contraction or dilatation of pupils, and coma. The patient must be carefully fed and nursed. *Canc.*, second dil., alt. *Scrof. 1*, second dil. in very frequent teaspoonfuls. Compress of *Canc. 5* alt. *Scrof.*. *White* or *Green* El. to head. *Blue* El. to temples, 18, 16, 17.

Spinal: Inflammation of the spinal pia mater which may be either tubercular or simple and of idiopathic origin. The former variety is often complicated with inflammation at the base of the brain. At first there are listlessness, chilliness, burning and boring pains in the back and pains extending round the body in girdle fashion. The skin becomes very sensitive to the touch. There is also retention of the fœces and urine. *Scrof 1*, second or third dil. alt. *Canc. 4*, second dil. alt. *Ang. 3*, second dil. *Canc. 5* ointment to spine.

Tubercular (cerebral) : An acute and very fatal febrile disease, commencing with malaise, vomiting, pains in the head, causing children when affected by the disease to start and cry out in their sleep. Afterwards the pupils of the eye become insensitive to light, the pulse-rate rises, and the heart becomes irregular. The child is quiet and drowsy or utters frequent plaintive cries. Stupor and coma follow. The only chance of cure is in the early stage of the disease. *Canc. 4*, second or third dil., alt. *Ang. 3*, second dil. Compress of *Canc. 1* alt. *Ang. 3* to head. 1 glob. *Scrof. 1* hourly.

Menstruation : The periodical discharge sometimes

takes place as often as once in twenty-one days, or as seldom as once in thirty-one days without any injury to health. The chief disorders affecting this function are :

1. *Amenorrhœa* : characterised by absence or deficiency of the discharge. This may arise from defective nutrition, phthisis, Bright's disease, or from abscess or disease of the ovaries or uterus. When arising from the latter causes, the disease is often incurable. In other cases the general health should be improved by means of *Canc. 5* alt. *Ang. 1* or *2*, first dil. 5 globs. *Scrof.* morning and at meals. Baths of *Canc. 5* alt. *Ang. 2*. *Red* El. to ovaries, 20, and dorsal spine.

2. *Dysmenorrhœa* : sharp pain accompanying the performance of the function, resulting from obstruction, disease of the uterus, &c. Rest in bed, hot baths, &c. are useful. In some cases surgical operations are necessary. 2 globs. *Scrof.* night and morning. *Ang. 1*, dil. alt. *Canc. 1*, second dil. A globule of *Canc. 1* (which greatly relieves pain) should be taken hourly for six hours if necessary. 5 globs. *Scrof.* at meals. Warm sitz baths of *Canc. 5* alt. *Ang. 3*. *Red* El. to 20.

Menstrual colic may be relieved by 2 or 3 globs. of *Canc.* every half-hour

3. *Menorrhagia* or *Menhorrhagia* : Flooding. The former term is applied to profuse menstruation ; the latter to hæmorrhage at other than the normal periods. Rest in bed, plugs of cotton wool saturated with *Ang. 1* and *Blue* El. *Ang. 3*, second dil., or *Ang. 1*, third dil. alt. *Canc. 1* or *Canc. 6*, second dil. *Ang. 3* ointment over cardiac region.

4. *Sudden suppression* : Give 5 globs. *Ang. 3* dry on

waking and alt. *Ang.* 3, first dil., with *Canc. 1*, first dil. Apply *Blue* El. to 20, 12. It is important to remember that the Angioticos in the first dil. tend to induce the menses, and in the second or third dil. to reduce them. The litre dil. has a neutral effect.

Mercurial Poisoning: The medicinal use of mercury often produces symptoms of acute or chronic poisoning. In acute cases there are burning in the throat, inflammation of the intestinal tract, vomiting, and whitening of the tongue. In chronic cases there commonly is salivation, and there often is a trembling resembling that of paralysis agitans. 5 globs. *Canc. 5* twice a day. *Scrof. 5* lit. dil. alt. *Canc. 1* lit. dil. In some cases, 1 glob. *Ven.* hourly.

Migraine or **Megrim** (Sick Headache): Periodical headache affecting one side of the head, preceded by disorders of sensation, and especially by a disturbance of vision. The patient sees a wavy glimmering. On the side of the head opposite to that on which this is first seen a boring pain is soon felt which spreads from this point and is followed by nausea. See Headache.

Miliaria: See Fevers.

Milk Crust: See Eczema. Give *Scrof.* to nurse.

Mortification: See Gangrene.

Mouth, bad taste in: *Scrof. 1* first dil. alt. *Canc. 1* first dil.; *Red* alt. *Yellow* El. to 5, 6. Gargles of *Red* or *White* El. *Feb. 1* pint dil. or 1 glob. in a wine glass taken in 3 doses at 10 minute intervals.

Mumps: An acute infectious disease which chiefly affects young people. At first there are malaise, chilliness and fever rising to 100° or 103°. The salivary glands, espacially the parotides, become enlarged. As a rule only one side of the face is affected. Sometimes, as the inflammation of the salivary glands declines, other parts, such as the mammæ or testicles, become affected. Rest in bed is generally advisable, especially if there is much fever. *Feb. 1* second dil. alt. *Canc. 1* second dil.; pour 5 drops of *White* El. on cranium; apply *Blue* El. to nape of neck; compress of *Canc.* 5; *Feb. 2* ointment to 24. *Lin.* ointment. Gargle of *White* El., 1 drachm to 5 oz. of water with or without glycerine.

Muscular atrophy: Progressive wasting of the muscular tissue, originating in alteration in the nerve centres. Treat like Marasmus.

Muscular Paralysis: See Paralysis.

Myalgia: Pain in a muscle. Treat as Rheumatism.

Myelitis: Inflammation of the spinal cord. See Spine.

Myocarditis: Inflammation of the wall of the heart. See Heart.

Myxœdema: This name was given by Dr. Ord to a progressive disease attacking women, in which, as he says, "the tissues of the body are invaded by a jelly-like, mucus-yielding dropsy, unaccompanied by albuminuria or other signs of primary affection of the kidneys." The patient's face is swollen, waxy-looking and anæmic. The expression becomes most sad. The skin everywhere is thickened, translucent, dry and rough. The hands become spade-like. The temperature of the body falls below normal. Vapour baths, careful diet, frictions of *Canc. 2* which should also be used internally in second dil. alt. *Feb. 1* second dil. *Ang. 3* third dil. Baths of *Canc. 5.*

Nævus: A congenital tumour composed of blood vessels. There are two varieties, of which the first is of a bright red colour, affecting only the cutaneous surfaces; and the second, which is seen through the skin, has a purplish tint, and may involve either the deeper structures of the body alone or both these and the skin. *Scrof. 1* should be given to infants, 1 glob. every 2 hours.

Nails, Diseases of: The chief inflammatory diseases affecting the nail are known as onychia and paronychia. The former term is applied to an inflammation involving the soft parts surrounding and beneath the nail, the latter to one affecting the walls of the nail. The internal use of *Scrof. 1*, with external applications of *Scrof. 5* may be recommended. When the diseases are associated with eczema, leprosy, scrofula, or syphilis, constitutional treatment adapted to these is of primary importance.

Nausea: This may be relieved by 5 to 8 globs. of *Scrof. 1* or *Scrof. Giap.* dry on the tongue or by *Scrof.* alt. *Canc. 1*, first dil. *Ang. 1* in the morning and *Feb. 1* at night will often relieve chronic nausea. Even in pregnancy these remedies are efficacious. In this condition, however, the second dil. of *Canc. 1* is better than the first. In the treatment of sea-sickness *Mal de mer* may be substituted for *Scrof.*

Necrosis: Death of the whole or part of a bone. *Canc. 4* or *3*, second or third dil., with *Ven.*, second or third dil. if syphilitic origin is suspected. Compresses of the same remedies. *Canc. 5* ointment to dorsal spine.

Nephritis: Inflammation of the kidney. See Kidney.

Nervous agitation: *Scrof. 1* third dil. alt. *Feb. 1*. *White* El. to 17. *Canc. 5* ointment to head. Baths of *Canc. 5* and *Scrof. 1*.

Nettle Rash: See Urticaria.

Neuralgia: Attacks of paroxysmal pain in the nerves. This may result from anything which lowers vitality or from gout, syphilis, dental caries, worms, or uterine disease. The pain is sometimes hammering, boring, or burning. The cause should be sought for and, if possible, removed. The remedies which are of greatest service in most cases are *Scrof. 1*, litre or first dil., local applications of *White* El., especially if the neuralgia is in the head or abdomen, or of *Red* alt. *Yellow* El. Compress of *White* El. alt. *Scrof.* or *Scrof. 5*. In syphilitic cases *Ven.*, second dil., and baths of *Ven.* alt. *Canc. 5* with *Feb. 2* alt. *Canc. 5* ointment to 24. In dental cases the mouth may be rinsed out with lotion of *Scrof.* alt. *Canc. 5*. In facial neuralgia which occurs periodically *Feb. 1*, second or third dil. alt. *Scrof.*, first or second dil., with *Red* or *White* El. to painful spots. If the neuralgia is congestive, *Ang. 3*, third dil., should take the place of *Scrof.*, and *Blue* El. be substituted for *Red* El. Ovarian neuralgia may result from anæmia or hysteria. When it does the cause must be attacked with *Scrof.*, second or third dil. or *Canc.*, second or third dil. If it occur at the periods, and is produced by congestion, *Ang. 1* must be given and frictions of *Blue* El. used. If worms cause the pain, *Ver.* is required. If malaria has been the originator, *Feb. 1* is needed, with *Feb. 2* to 24. In hypochondriacal cases also the two latter remedies must be used.

Neuritis: Inflammation of a nerve. *Scrof. 1* second or third dil., with local applications of *White* or *Red* El.

Nose, *Bleeding from*: See Epistaxis.

" *Polypus in*: See Polypus

Nostalgia: Home Sickness. Treat like Melancholia.

Nymphomania: *Canc. 2* second dil. *White* El. to back of neck, 17, 18, and 20. Baths of *Canc. 5*. Ointment of *Canc. 5* to 20, 22.

Obesity: Excessive corpulence may be diminished by abstinence from starchy foods, and by considerably diminishing the quantity of fluid taken. Exercise is very beneficial. *Scrof. 1* or *Canc. 4* first dil.; 5 globs. *Scrof.* at meals. Women often need *Canc. 1* second dil. or *Canc. 4* second dil. in alternation with *Scrof.* Baths of *Scrof. 1* or *Ang. 2*. In some cases the addition of *Ven.* has been found useful.

Œsophagitis: Inflammation of the tube connecting the pharynx with the stomach. At first there is burning or lancinating pain, sometimes inducing vomiting. The pain is much aggravated by swallowing. *Scrof. 1* first or second dil. *Red* El. to 5, 17, 18. Warm fomentations or compresses of *Scrof. 5* and *Red* El., or *Scrof. 5* ointment,

Onychia: See Nails.

Ophthalmia: See Eyes.

Orchitis: Inflammation of the testes. *Scrof. 1* or *2* litre dil. *Scrof. 5* alt. *Ang. 3* baths. If syphilitic add *Ven.* internally and externally.

Osteitis: Inflammation of bone. See Bones.

Otitis: Inflammation of the Ear. See Ear.

Otorrhœa: Discharge from the Ear. See Ear.

Ovarian Neuralgia: See Neuralgia.

Ovaritis: Inflammation of the Ovaries. The acute form is marked by pain over the pubes, and tenderness of one iliac region. Acute cases are characterised by paroxysms of pain at the periods. *Scrof. 1* second or third dil. alt. *Canc. 1* second dil. or 1 glob. *Canc. 5* hourly. *Canc. 1* or *5* compress and ointment over the ovaries. 3 drops of *Blue* El. *Red* alt. *Yellow* El. to 18, 20, and sides of spine.

Ozœna: A disease resulting from syphilis, struma, necrosis of bones, &c., characterised by ulceration in, and a fœtid, chronic discharge from, the nose. *Scrof. 1* second second dil. and in aspirations. If this does not suffice, *Scrof. 1* second dil. alt. *Canc.* second dil. or *Canc.* second dil. alt. *Ven.* second dil. if syphilitic origin is suspected. Comp. of *Green* El. to root of Nose. Syringe the nose with warm salted water medicated with *Canc. 5* and *Green* El. Alt. *Scrof. 1* and *Canc. 5* ointment to base of nose. Applications of *Red* alt. *Yellow* El. to 1, 5, 18, 17.

Pain is experienced when the nerve centres undergo certain abnormal perturbations. It often happens that the pain is felt at a nerve centre far removed from the producing cause of the disturbance. It will be useful to remember that continuous dull frontal headache may be caused by gastric derangement; severe pain at the back of the head often accompanies Bright's disease; violent, crushing headaches may be dependent upon syphilis; shooting pains in the head may be due to locomotor ataxy; the feeling as if a nail were being driven into the head may accompany hysteria; pain in the chest-wall may be due to rheumatic neuralgia, the pressure of an aneurism, or syphilitic periostitis; dull pain in the heart may be caused by nervous debility; sharp pain under the breast, accompanied by palpitation may be hysterical; the feeling as if the heart had been grasped with an iron hand is symptomatic of angina pectoris; pain in the spinal column may result from nervous exhaustion; acute pain in the abdomen may be produced by strangulated hernia; severe paroxysmal pain on one side of the loins may be caused by stone in the kidney; pain in the back may be dependent upon flatulent distention of the bowels or upon abscess in the rectum; lightning-like pains in the limbs may mark the early stage of locomotor ataxy. In all these cases the treatment must be directed to the cause of pain, and suitable applications made to the affected nerve centres. Should this not succeed at first, *Ang.* should be applied in compresses or ointments to prepare the way for them. This is specially the case in the treatment of rheumatic gout and sciatica. It is impossible to give more than a few hints. *Red* El. is useful in rheumatic pains; *White* and *Yellow* El. in neuralgic pains; *Green* El. in articular or lancinating pains, especially in the pains of cancer; *Blue* El. in burning cancer pains. The application of *Blue* El. or of *Red* alt. *Yellow* El., according to the temperament, to the chief nerve centres is often useful in combating pain. Baths of *Canc. 5* and compress and ointment of the same remedy are also valuable. Nocturnal osseous pains should be treated with *Ven.* second dil. alt. *Ang.* second dil.; with 5 globs *Canc.* night and morning, and 5 globs. *Scrof.* at meals. Pains in the left side, arising from heart affections, should be treated with *Ang. 3* third dil., and compress of *Ang. 3* to heart; with *Blue* El. to 18. Pains on the right side, arising from liver disease, should be treated with *Feb. 1* second or lit. dil. and *Feb. 2* ointment to 24.

Palpitation: Pass a few drops of *Blue* El. lightly over the heart. (See Heart.)

Palsy: See Paralysis.

Pancreatitis: Inflammation of the pancreas. The symptoms of acute pancreatitis include deep-seated pain in the epigastrium and some feverishness, nausea, vomiting, thirst, constipation, rapid breathing, weak pulse. The chronic form of the disease presents less marked symptoms, and is difficult to diagnose. *Scrof. 1* second dil. alt. *Feb. 1* second dil. *Red* alt. *Yellow* El. to 18. Ointment of *Feb. 2* to 24.

Paralysis: Loss of motor or sensory power. Motor paralysis may result from disease of the brain, spinal cord, nerve centres, or peripheral nerves. A variety of paralysis known as the "hysterical" arises simply from functional perversion. Paralysis originating in the brain usually begins with an attack of apoplexy or epilepsy or with a series of these, and is ordinarily confined to half the body (Hemiplegia). Paralysis originating in the spinal column commonly affects both sides, and is accompanied with a feeling as if a girdle were fastened round the body at the junction of the parts affected with those not affected. Paralysis originating in disease or injury of particular nerve trunks only produces loss of power in the muscles governed by those nerves. An obscure and but little understood form of paralysis known as *paralysis agitans*, sometimes affects the nerve centres of aged people. Paralytic affections, usually of a peripheral origin, sometimes accompany diphtheria and other zymotic diseases. A thickening of the speech usually forms the earliest indication of their approach. The voice sinks to a whisper and becomes markedly nasal. The eyelids droop. The intestinal canal and bladder are often paralysed.

When there are indications of approaching paralysis,

give 10 to 20 globs. of *Scrof.* 1 dry on the tongue; apply *Red* El. to the six chief nerve centres, and bathe the head with *White* El. Or if there are congestive symptoms, give *Ang.* 2 second dil.; apply *Blue* El. to nerves of head, and especially to temples, 17, 18; gently rub *Ang.* 3 ointment over heart, and give 5 to 10 drops of *Blue* El.

In paralysis originating in the brain and affecting half the body give *Ang.* 3, 2 or 1, second or third dil. 5 or 10 drops of *Blue* El. twice a day, and apply *Blue* El. to the chief points, and along the spine. The same internal treatment should be used in all cases where persons of sanguine temperament are attacked.

In paralysis originating in the spine: *Scrof.*, second or third dil. alt. *Canc.*, second or third dil. are best for persons of lymphatic temperament and *Ang.*, second or third dil. alt. *Canc.*, second or third dil., for those of sanguine temperament.

In paralysis of peripheral origin (including diptheritic paralysis): *Scrof.*, second or third dil., should be given to lymphatic patients; *Ang.*, second or third dil., to sanguine patients; and these remedies alternated to those of mixed temperaments. Suitable compresses, &c., may be used, such as, in paralysis of bladder: compress of *White* El. to 20, 22, 25. Ointment of *Canc.* 5 alt. *Scrof.* alt. *Ang.* 3 to the pubes, and injections of *White* El. In congestive paralysis of tongue *Ang.* 3 ointment to hypoglossi, and gargles of *Ang.* 3 and *Blue* El. In paralysis of eyelids compress of *Canc.* 5, *White* or *Blue* El.; ointment of *Scrof.* 5 and *Ang.* 3. In nervous paralysis of tongue apply *Red* alt. *Yellow* El. to 16, 18, 17. *Canc.* 5 ointment to 16; gargles of *Scrof.* 1, *Canc.* 5 and *White* El. In facial paralysis compress of *White* El. and ointment of *Canc. 5* to part affected, and to the whole head. In general hemiplegia compress of *Ang. 3*; light application of *Blue* El. to nerves of head and to spine; and of *White* El. to other chief centres.

Paronychia (Whitlow): See Nails, diseases of.

Parotitis: See Mumps.

Pellagra: An erythematous skin disease chiefly affecting the back of the hands, the neck and the head, accompanied by grave constitutional disorders, marked by nausea, diarrhœa, neuralgic pains, prostration, &c. Patients should feed well and avoid exposure to the sun. *Scrof.* or *Canc.*, third dil., alt. *Ang. 3*, second dil.

Pericarditis, Inflammation of the pericardium: See Heart.

Periostitis: Inflammation of the periosteum. See Bones.

Peritonitis: Inflammation of the peritoneum, the chief serous membrane of the body. The acute form may arise from injury, perforation, rupture, direct irritation, or the extension of neighbouring inflammations, especially in the case of women, as the peritoneum is directly connected with the uterus through the fallopian tubes. Its chief symptoms are severe pain, at first local, and then extending over the whole of the abdomen, and leading the patient to lie on the back with the thighs and knees bent and the legs well drawn up. The abdomen becomes much distended and exquisitely tender. The appetite is lost. Thirst is intense. A disagreeable taste is experienced. As a rule there is obstinate constipation. The cause of the inflammation must be sought for and, if possible, removed.

For the first hour or two give *Scrof. 1*, first dil. alt. *Feb. 1* first, litre, or second dil., according to the amount of feverishness. Compresses of *Canc. 5*. Afterwards give *Canc. 1*, second dil. alt. with *Feb. 1* if the fever continue; globs. *Scrof. 1* morning and evening. Frequently changed cold abdominal compress of *Canc. 5*, alt. *Ang. 3* alt. *White* El.; *Feb. 2* compress or ointment to 24 Should the patient become delirious apply *Red* El. to 17 and compress of *Canc. 5* to the head. The patient should be kept at rest in bed and means used to prevent the bed-clothes from pressing on the abdomen. It is sometimes advisable to substitute warm compresses for cold ones as the disease progresses. Liquid food only should be given. If there is any vomiting give 5 globs. *Scrof. Giap.* For chronic forms of the disease give *Canc. 1* or *5*, second or third dil. in morning, *Yellow* El. afternoon, alt. *Feb. 1*, third dil. at night. An occasional dry glob. of *Ang. 3* should be given if there is any intestinal hæmorrhage.

Perspiration, excessive: *Scrof. 1*, first or litre dil. *Red* alt. *Yellow* or *White* to 5, 18, 17. Baths of *Canc. 5* *Scrof.* or *White* El.

Pharyngitis: A non-exudative catarrhal inflammation of the pharynx, the catarrh extending from the back of the nostrils to the gullet. At first there may be feverishness. The voice becomes husky and nasal. Abundant mucus is secreted. At the outset the patient should be confined to bed and given *Feb. 1*, first dil. After a short time, if the first named remedy does not suffice to subdue the disease, *Scrof. 1*, first or litre dil. should be taken. A few teaspoonfuls daily of *Feb. 1*, second dil. Gargles of *Scrof. 1*. Milk in abundance may be given.

Warm fomentations or a compress of *Domfin* or *Canc. 5*. Gargles of *Pet. 1* with *White* El. and glycerine.

Phlebitis: Inflammation of a vein. *Ang. 1* first or second dil. Compress of *Ang. 3* or *Blue* El. on the diseased veins. *Ang. 3* ointment to heart. Baths of *Ang. 2* or *Blue* El. (1 tablespoonful to a bathful of water).

Phlegmasia Alba Dolens: White Leg. A disease which chiefly attacks lying-in women. After a short season of pain, a hard elastic swelling appears in one part of the leg and spreads upwards or downwards until the whole limb is affected, and becomes pale and glossy. *Canc. 1*, second dil. alt. *Ang.*, second dil. *Canc. 5* alt. *Ang. 3* ointment gently applied to, but not rubbed on, the swollen member.

Phthisis: See Consumption.

Piles: See Hæmorrhoids.

Pityriasis: A scurfy or scaly skin disease, accompanied with heat and redness, but with no exudation. *Scrof. 1* or *5*, second or third dil. Baths of *Scrof. 1* or *5*.

Pleurisy: Inflammation of the membrane which surrounds the lungs, accompanied by interstitial effusion. It may be caused by local injury, the contact of irritating substances, a rheumatic or gouty habit, a chill, or may occur as a complication of pneumonia, kidney diseases, blood-poisoning, &c. At the outset there are lancinating stabbing pains below the nipple, on one side of the body, which are increased by coughing, by pressure, or by taking a deep breath. On applying the ear or the stethoscope to the affected part of the chest during the first stage of the disease, a peculiar friction sound may be heard. There is a short frequent cough. The face is flushed.

The urine is scanty and high-coloured. *Feb. 1*, second dil. alt. *Scrof. 1*, second dil., alt. *Pet. 1* or *2*, second dil. *Canc. 5* ointment to chest; *Feb. 2* ointment to 24; *White* El. to 5, 18, 17.

Pleurodynia: Muscular rheumatism or cramp affecting the chest wall. For treatment see Cramp and Rheumatism.

Podagra: See Gout.

Poisoning: This may result from the action of (1.) *Corrosives*, including mineral acids, such as hydrochloric, nitric, oxalic and sulphuric; caustic alkalies such as potash, soda and ammonia; or salts, such as nitrate of silver, potassium bisulphate, &c. (2.) *Irritants*, such as arsenic, salts of antimony, essential oils and cantharides, or (3.) *Neurotics* such as opium, morphia, digitalis, prussic acid, belladonna, alcohol, &c. The corrosives immediately produce burning sensations in the alimentary canal, vomiting (in most cases), and distension of the abdomen. Irritant poisons take longer in producing symptoms of poisoning. These include burning pain in the throat and epigastrium, nausea, vomiting, abdominal distension and diarrhœa. Neurotic poisons cause varying symptoms. Aconite produces a peculiar numbness and tingling of the skin. Carbolic acid whitens the membrane which it touches and blackens the urine. Morphia and opium contract the pupils of the eye, bring on a comatose sleep, and suppress the secretions. Prussic acid originates convulsions, greatly disturbs the breathing, and dilates the pupils of the eyes. In cases of poisoning by corrosive acids lime water, chalk, or whitening are useful antidotes. The harmful effects of the caustic alkalies may be lessened by taking highly diluted acid liquids. In both these cases emetics of mustard and water may be taken. An emetic should be given immediately after the first symptoms of poisoning appear. After prussic acid poisoning cold water should be poured over the head, neck and down the spine. *Red* El. should be applied to 5, 6, 18, the crown of the head and to the spine. Artificial respiration must be resorted to. Stimulants should be given. Not a moment should be lost. After narcotic poisoning the stomach pump should, if possible, be used, or an emetic be given; strong black coffee (but no wine or brandy) should be given, and the patient kept walking. On no account must he be allowed to sleep. If necessary, cold water must be dashed into his face, pins must be stuck into him, and he must be kept walking for hours. After poisoning by corrosive sublimate the patient should take an emetic and then swallow the contents of several eggs, or flour and water, or milk. In any of these cases the nearest medical man should be summoned without delay.

It may be noted that one of the deadliest of poisons, viz., prussic acid is frequently present in almond flavouring, and that a number of deaths have occurred through the use of this in the preparation of food.

The after effects of poisoning may be counteracted by 10 globs. of *Scrof. 1* dry followed by *Scrof. 5* first dil. Applications of *Red* alt. *Yellow* El. to 5, 17, 18, and baths of *Scrof. 1* alt. *Scrof. 5*.

Polypus: A pedunculated growth rooted in a mucous surface, such as the mucous membrane of the bladder, the ear, the gums, the larynx, the intestines, the nose, the palate, the vulva or the uterus. *Scrof. 1* alt. *Canc. 4*, or

Canc. 4 alt. *Ven.* Compresses, injections, or inhalations (according to the part affected) of *Canc. 5* or *Canc. 4.* When the polypus is in the palate or larynx use gargles of *Canc. 1* alt. *Canc. 5*, alt. *Green* or *White* El.

Polyuria (Diabetes insipidus): Excessive flow of watery non-albuminous urine which is of low specific gravity (from 1·001 to 1·008 or 1·010). *Scrof. 1* first or lit. dil. Compress of *Red* El. alt. *Scrof. 1* on the kidney region, or *Lin.* ointment alt. with *Scrof. 5* ointment.

Pregnancy: During the whole time take *Scrof. 1* first or lit. dil., and frequent sitz-baths.

Prolapsus Ani: falling of the Anus. *Scrof.* or *Canc. 1* or *5* or *Ver.;* compress of *Canc. 5* or *Scrof. 5; Red* alt. *Yellow* El. to 20, 22; sitz-baths of *Canc. 5;* injections of *White* El.

Prolapsus Uteri: Falling of the Womb. See Womb.

Prostration: *Scrof. 1* first or lit. dil,; *Red* El. to 6, nerves of head and sides of spine; baths of *Canc. 1* or *5*, or *Lin.*

Prostatitis: Inflammation of the prostate. It may be acute or chronic. *Scrof. 1* or *5* second or third dil. alt. *Canc. 6* second dil.; compress of *Canc. 5* to the perineum; hot sitz-baths of *Canc. 5* alt. *Lin.*

Proud Flesh: *Ang. 1* or *2* second dil.; compress of *Scrof. 5* alt. *Ang. 3.*

Prurigo: A skin disease characterised by peculiarly pungent itching, accompanied with a sensation resembling the creeping of animals through the skin. It chiefly occurs in the aged. *Scrof. 1* second or third dil. Baths or sitz-baths of *Canc. 5.* Russian baths are also valuable.

Pruritus: Itching of the skin of the external parts of mucous membranes. *Scrof. 1* second or third dil. alt. *Ang. 3* second dil. Baths of *Canc. 5* alt. *Scrof. 1* alt. *Ang. 3*. *Scrof. 5* baths or ointment, sometimes *Ver.*

Psoriasis: Lepra vulgaris. A skin disease characterized by dry whitish silvery scales and cracking of the skin. *Scrof. 1* or *5* third dil. alt. *Ang. 1* or *3* second dil. alt. *Feb. 1* litre dil.; warm baths of *Scrof. 1* or *Lin.* In some cases *Scrof. 5* ointment.

Pustules, malignant: *Canc. 1* second dil. alt. *Ang. 3* second dil. *Canc. 5* ointment.

Puerperal Fever: *Scrof. 1* second dil. alt. *Feb. 1* second or third dil. alt. *Canc. 1* second dil.

Pyæmia: Blood poisoning, through the entrance of decomposing animal matter into the blood. The symptoms include rigors, pains in the limbs, intermittent fever, dry brown tongue, depression, and, in the least acute cases, swelling of joints or formation of abscesses or pustules. Strong dose of *Scrof. 5* (5 globs. to 6 ounces of water) alt. with *Canc. 5* first dil. alt. *Ang. 2* first dil. *Feb. 2* ointment to 24. Watch the effect of each dose in urgent cases, and act accordingly.

Quinsy: See Tonsillitis.

Rectum, Cancer in. See Cancer.

Rectum, Falling of: Protrusion of a portion of the bowel. The protruded part may be put back by means of the well-oiled fore-finger. Compresses of *Canc. 4*. *Canc. 1* second dil. Enemata with *Blue* or *White* El.

Rectum, Polypus of: See Polypus.

Relapsing Fever: See Fever.

Remittent Fever. See Fever.

Renal Calculus: See Calculus.

Resuscitation: The following are the chief rules for the restoration of the apparently dead: (1) if from Apoplexy or Sunstroke, raise the head; apply cold water compresses to it; remove tight clothing. (2) If from Drowning or Suffocation, or Narcotic Poisoning: all tight clothing should be removed, the mouth should be cleansed and the tongue kept drawn forward by means of an elastic band, and 8 or 10 dry globs. of *Scrof. 1* put on it. The patient should be laid on his back with his head slightly raised. His arms should then be grasped just above the elbows and drawn gently and steadily upwards till they meet above the head, in order to imitate the chest movement which takes place in the act of inspiration. The arms should then be turned down and pressed gently and firmly for two seconds against the chest in order to press air out of the lungs, as in the natural act of expiration. The operation will be rendered easier if, when the patient's arms are turned down, an assistant press together the lower part of the ribs and diaphragm with both hands laid flat upon these. The act of artificial inspiration should be repeated fifteen times a minute until natural breathing begins, when the patient should be wrapped up in dry blankets and well rubbed. *Red* El. and hot bottles, &c., may be applied to the soles, armpits, pit of stomach, and between the thighs. After the recovery of consciousness give *Scrof. 1*, first dil.

Retention of Urine: See Urine.

Rheumatic Gout: *Canc. 1*, second dil; *Canc. 5* lotion and baths; *Green* El. to joints. See also Gout.

Rheumatism, Acute: See Fevers.

Chronic: a disease which often follows acute rheumatism, and, like it, is traceable to a constitutional cachexia. It is because the blood contains a morbid product that the pain, stiffness and swelling appear. Dyspeptic symptoms are generally marked. The pains of rheumatism may generally be relieved by *Red* alt. *Yellow* El. and by *Scrof. 5* ointment, if the rheumatism affect the muscles, or by *Green* El. if it affect the joints. Internally *Scrof. 1*, second dil., if there be no crisis, or *Scrof. 1* third dil. if there be a crisis. Flannel should be worn next the skin by those afflicted with rheumatism.

Rickets: A disease which is closely allied to scrofula, if it be not one form of it. The bones of its victims are deficient in earthy phosphates. Curvature of the spine or bow-leggedness result from this. The other symptoms include profuse perspiration from the upper part of the body, large appetite, irregular bowels, drowsiness in the daytime and restlessness at night. The head of a ricketty child is large, flattened, and slow in closing. The face is small, the abdomen is large, and the chest narrow and prominent. *Scrof. 1*, litre dil. alt. *Canc. 4*, litre dil.; 3 to 5 globs. *Scrof.* at meals. *Red* alt. *Yellow* El. to 5, 6, 18, 17, and to parts affected. Baths of *Scrof. 1* alt. *Scrof. 5*, alt. *Canc. 5*. *Canc. 5* ointment to whole head.

Ringworm: a fungus parasite consisting of oval spores about $\frac{1}{1000}$ inch in diameter, which occurs in circular patches on the scalp, the beard or the body. *Scrof. 5* ointment, alt. *Canc. 5* ointment with *Scrof. 1* internally. Give *Scrof. 1* alt. *Canc. 1* in dil. Baths and compresses of *Scrof. 5*, *Canc. 5*, or *Lin.* The general health may be improved by means of *Scrof.*

Rupture (Hernia): *Scrof. 1* dil. Compress of *Red* El. and *Lord. Lord* ointment.

Salivation: Children should have *Ver.*, second dil. with compress and ointment of *Canc. 5* to 24. Adults require *Scrof.* alt. *Ven.* first dil. Gargles of *White* El. and *Canc. 5*.

St. Vitus' Dance: See Chorea.

Scabies (Itch): a contagious skin disease of a very irritating character. A minute parasite produces an eruption of small transparent vesicles chiefly on the thin skin in the flexures of the joints and in other delicate parts. *Scrof. 1* in litre or second dil. and *Scrof. 5* ointment will free the system from this troublesome complaint. While it lasts care must be taken to disinfect the clothes worn by the patient. Contaminated linen should be immersed in boiling water. Other clothes should be ironed with a hot iron, or hung in hot air at a temperature of 170°.

Scald Head: *Scrof.* dil. or *Scrof.* alt. *Canc.* Baths of *Scrof. 1* or *5* alt. *Lin.* Compress of *Scrof. 5* or *Canc. 5*, *White* or *Red* El.

Scarlatina. See Fevers.

Sciatica: Neuralgia of the great sciatic nerve. It may arise from exposure to cold or wet, or from rheumatism, or may be a complication of gout, or of biliary calculus. Rub *Yellow* El. over the joint where the pain is most severe and *Red* El. on hollow of foot. In very severe cases the hypodermic injection of *White* El. may be tried near nerve points. In some instances and *Red* alt. *Yellow* to sacral nerves. Sanguine temperaments require *Blue* El., *Ang. 2* compress and ointment. When there is biliary calculus apply compress of *White* El. to the three sciatic points, and *Red* alt. *Yellow* El. to same. *Feb. 1*, second dil. alt. with *Scrof. 2* first dil.

Scrofula (King's Evil): A tendency to the deposition of tubercles and, therefore, to pulmonary phthisis. Glandular swellings, inflammations of the joints, ulcers in the cornea, chronic abscesses are common results of the presence of this tendency. Scrofulous children are often pigeon-breasted, with enlarged abdomen, languid circulation, furred tongue and fœtid breath. *Scrof. 1* lit. dil. alt. *Canc.* or sometimes *Ven.* in deep-seated cases. *Red* alt. *Yellow* El. to 5, 18, 17. Baths of *Scrof.* alt. *Canc. 5* or *Ven.* Nutritious articles of diet, and especially eggs and milk are of great service. Regular open-air exercise and sea-bathing are useful.

Scurf in Head: *Scrof.* or sometimes *Canc.*; *Scrof. 5* ointment. If irritation and redness precede the scurf, *Ang. 2* ointment, followed by *Canc. 5* and *Scrof. 5* ointment.

Scurvy (Scorbutus): A vitiation of the blood, producing a tendency to hæmorrhage and congestion, especially in the gums. The patient is seized with languor, depression of spirits, &c. *Scrof. 5* or *Scrof. 2* or *Canc. 1* alt *Ang. 3* second dil; *Canc. 5* alt. *Scrof. 5* over open bleeding surface; baths of *Lin.*; *Ang 3* to 27; *Feb. 2* to 24; gargles of *Blue* El.; 2 to 5 drops of *Blue* El.

Sea-sickness: To prevent: Take litre or first dil. of *Anti-mal-de-mer* or of *Scrof. Giap.* a day before sailing. During the voyage take first or second dil. *Anti-mal-de-mer*, and put 5 to 8 globs. of this remedy dry on the tongue whenever a sensation of nausea is experienced. A cold compress of spongio-piline, saturated with a lotion of 4 globs of *Anti-mal-de-mer* and 4 drops of *White* El. to each ounce of water, may be worn over stomach and renewed when dry.

Septicæmia: Blood poisoning. For treatment see Pyæmia.

Serpentine Crusts: See Syphilis.

Shingles: See Herpes.

Sick Headache: *Scrof. Giap.* and *Verm.* See Migraine.

Skin Diseases: For most of these *Scrof. 1* or *5* should be used. As a rule a high dilution (the second or third) is needed. Stronger doses increase the eruption. For round red patches, *Ang. 1* alt. *Scrof. 5.*

Skin, Spots on: *Scrof. 1* second dil. or *Scrof. 5* second dil.; compress of *Canc. 5* or *Feb. 2* to 24; *Red* alt. *Yellow* El. to 5, 18, 17; *Canc. 5* alt. *Scrof. 1* baths; *Feb. 2* and *Canc. 5* ointment to 24.

Skin, Liver Spots: *Feb. 1* second dil.; *White* El. to 24; *Feb. 2* alt. *Canc. 5* ointment to 24; baths of *Canc. 5.*

Skin, Wine-coloured Spots: *Ang. 1* or *2* second dil.; baths and compress of *Blue* El. or *Ang. 3;* ointment of *Ang. 3, Canc. 5.*

Skin, Ulceration of: *Canc.* litre dil. alt. *Scrof. 5* litre dil.; compresses of *Scrof. 5* alt. *Canc. 5; White* or *Blue* El. Applications of *Red* alt. *Yellow* El. to 5, 18, 17.; *Feb. 2* ointment to 24; baths of *Canc. 5* alt. *Ang. 2.*

Sleeplessness: If arising from a febrile state of the blood, give 2 globs. *Feb. 1* dry at night, and a warm bath of *Feb. 2* at night. If from congestive tendency, a globule of *Ang. 3* should be taken on retiring. If from nervous exhaustion, a globule or two of *Scrof. 1.* At night take a warm bath of *Scrof. 1.* To children give 2 globs. *Ver.* night and morning.

Small-pox : *Scrof. 1*, alt. *Feb. 1.* See Fevers.

Smell, Loss of: *Scrof. 1* first dil.; compress of *Canc. 5* or *Scrof.; Blue* El. or *Red* alt. *Yellow* El. to root of nose. Inhalations of *Scrof. 5*; ointment of *Canc. 5* alt. *Scrof.* alt. *Ang. 2.*

Snake Bites : *Canc. 1* first dil. alt. *Ang. 3* third dil.

Somnambulism : a state in which a patient goes about with at least the greater part of his faculties in a state of sleep or unconsciousness. It is usually associated with nervous diseases. *Scrof. 1*, third dil. alt. *Feb. 1*, second dil. *White* El. to 17. *Feb. 2* ointment to 24. Women require *Canc. 1*, second dil., or *Canc. 5*, second dil., instead of *Scrof.*

Spasms : 5 globs. *Scrof.* dry on tongue. If from worms *Ver.* in litre dil. *Ver. 2* ointment over abdomen. Enemata of *Yellow* El. and *Ver. 2.*

Spasms of Womb : *Canc. 2*, second dil. *Red* alt. *Yellow* El. to 18, 6, 5, 20, 22.

Speech, Difficulty of: Apply *Red* alt. *Yellow* El. to 9, 13, 18, 17. *Canc.* ointment to 9, 13. Use gargles of *Red* or *White* El. and *Scrof. 1.*

Spermatorrhœa : This ailment frequently follows the practice of self-abuse, a practice which is fearfully common, and which works enormous havoc among the young of both sexes. Mistaken modesty prevents parents and teachers from giving children warnings against this most injurious vice, similar to those which they address to them with reference to drinking, gambling, &c. Hence many are completely caught in its fateful snares ere they are aware that there is anything morally or physically evil in it. No parent should send a child to school, and especially to a boarding school, without plainly pointing out to him the danger of being led to form the habit. Among its consequences may be mentioned nervous prostration, loss of flesh, palpitation, loss of memory, low-spiritedness, bashfulness, indecision, pains in the back, digestive derangement, &c. Not the least of the evils is the difficulty of abandoning the habit when once it has been acquired. It is only after a long and severe struggle, sometimes prolonged over years, that some are able to shake themselves free from its snares. And even then the physical consequences remain. To remedy these give *Scrof. 1*, litre or second dil., sometimes third dil.; 3 to 5 globs. *Scrof. 1* at meals. Apply *Red* alt. *Yellow* El. to 5, 6, 12, 17, 18, and *White* El. to 20, 22, 25, and *Ang. 3* ointment to heart. Drops of *Blue* El. Cool baths of *Scrof. 1* alt. *Ang. 3.* Sitz-baths of *Lin.*

Spinal Curvature: The spinal column may be curved angularly or laterally. Angular curvature is due to caries of the anterior bone or cartilage. Lateral curvature may be produced by bad postures. The former generally occurs in subjects of scrofula. *Scrof. 1*, second dil.; 5 globs. *Lin.* at meals; *Scrof. 5* lotion along the spine. In a two ounce bottle, dissolve 30 to 40 globs. of *Scrof. 5* in half a teaspoonful of *White* or *Red* El. Add half-an-ounce of glycerine. Shake well and fill up with water. Begin with *White* El., afterwards use *Red* El. *Red* alt. *Yellow* to 6, 12, 18, 5, and along the dorsal spine.

Lateral curvation may be treated with the same remedies. Hurtful postures must be carefully avoided. Good diet, pure air, and suitable gymnastic exercises are important.

Spinal Inflammation (Myelitis): *Scrof. 1*, second dil., alt. *Canc. 1*, second dil. The Electricities are not to be used before convalescence. *Canc. 5* ointment over the head. During convalescence *Red* alt. Yellow El. may be applied to 5, 6, 7, 17, 18, and to the entire spine.

Spina Ventosa: Painful dilatation of bone tissues. *Canc. 4*, second dil., alt. *Ang. 1*, second dil. *Green* El. *Canc. 5* baths.

Spitting of Blood: See Hæmoptysis.

Sores (ordinary): *Scrof. 1* first dil., or, if extensive and deep, *Scrof. 1* lit. dil. alt. *Canc. 1* lit. dil. To relieve pain, apply compresses of *Green* El. and *Canc. 1*. If there is hæmorrhage, compresses of *Ang. 2* and *Blue* El. For sore legs use *Scrof. 1* lotion (3 globs. to the ounce). In many cases lotions or compresses of *Scrof. 1*, *Ang. 2* and *Canc. 1* may be alternated. The *Scrof.* rouses the lymphatics, the *Ang.* gives tone to the blood-vessels, and the *Canc.* assists the expulsion of the effete matter.

Spleen: This organ is greatly enlarged in intermittent fevers and in leucocythemia. It is also liable to waxy degeneration, &c. For all diseases of the spleen *Feb. 1* lit. or second dil. is the great remedy; with *Feb. 2* ointment to 24; *Feb. 2* compress to 24. Sometimes a stronger dose of *Feb.* may be given. In cases of splenitis, add *Scrof. 5* second dil. and *Red* alt. *Yellow* El. to 5, 18. Baths of *Canc. 5* or *White* El.

Splinters: After extracting the splinter with forceps, or fingers or with sponge and water, if the wound is lacerated, steep the part in a warm bath, medicated with 25 drops of *Blue* El. to each six ounces of water (three-quarters tumblerful). If there is any difficulty in extracting the splinter, apply, for an hour, a warm compress and *Scrof. 1*, covered with oiled silk.

Sprains: Give 2 globs. *Scrof. 1* twice a day. *Red* alt. *Yellow* El. to 5, 18, 17 and nerves of part; *Scrof. 5.* If swollen or inflamed, *Ang. 3* ointment alt. *Scrof. 5* ointment.

Stammering: *Scrof. 1* lit or second dil.; *Red* or *Yellow* El. to 16; *Canc. 5* to 16; gargles of *Red* or *White* El. It is a good praetice to beat time as the words are spoken.

Staphyloma: See Eye.

Sterility, In man: *Scrof. 1* first dil.; in woman, *Canc.* second or third dil. alt. *Scrof.* second or third dil. For either, 5 globs. *Scrof. 1* at meals; *Canc. 5* ointment to sacrum.

Stiff Neck (Crick in the Neck): Rheumatism in the muscles of the neck. Treat like Rheumatism.

Stings of Insects: *Canc. 1* lit. dil. Compresses of *Canc. 5* or *Lin.* alt. *Scrof.*; applications of *Red*, *White* or *Blue* El. *Lin.* or *Scrof. 5* ointment.

Stitch in Side: *Scrof. 1* first dil. *Red* alt. *Yellow* El. to 7.

Stomach, Cancer in: See Cancer.

Stomach, Dilatation of: *Scrof. 1* or *2.* Sometimes it is best to give 5 globs. of *Scrof. 2*, followed in twenty minutes by 5 globs. *Ver. 1.* *White* El. to 12, 17; *Feb. 2* ointment to 24.

Stomach, Gastralgia: Sharp burning pains in the

stomach, accompanied by distension, eructations, and often by nausea. One form of it results from ancient syphilitic taint, and is attended by periodical vomiting. *Scrof. 1* first dil.; *Red* alt. *Yellow* El. to 6; *Feb. 2* alt. *Canc. 5* to 24. If resulting from syphilitic taint, give *Feb 1* lit. dil. alt. *Ven.* lit. dil.

Stomach, Cancer at upper orifice of: *Canc. 1* second dil.; compresses of *White* El.; *Red* alt. *Yellow* El. to 5, 18, 17. Ointment of *Canc. 5* to the stomach region, and *Feb. 2* to 24. See Cancer.

Stomatitis: Inflammation of the mouth. There are red patches on the lining of the mouth, from which a fluid exudes. *Scrof. 1* lit. or second dil. Wash out the mouth with *Scrof. 1* or *5* or *Lin.* lotion.

Stone: See Calculus.

Straining at Stool: See Tenesmus.

Stricture: Compress of *Canc. 5* alt. *Ang. 3.* and ointments of the same remedies.

Stricture of Urethra: This may be organic or spasmodic. Organic stricture may result from inflammation excited either by gonorrhœa or by injury. Spasmodic stricture may result from abnormal muscular action or from local congestion or inflammation. There is pain in the canal when water is passed. The stream is flattened and diminished in volume. Subsequently the urine becomes alkaline and ropy. *Scrof. 1* lit. dil.; compress of *White* El.; warm baths of *Scrof. 1*; rectal injections of *Canc. 5* alt. *Ang. 3.*

Struma: See Scrofula.

Stupor through abuse of Quinine: 2 or 3 globs. of *Scrof. 1* or *5* three times a day. *Scrof. 5* alt. *Ang. 2* ointment to head and spine. *Feb. 1* dil.

Suicidal Tendency: Treat like Melancholia.

Sunstroke (Heat Apoplexy. Heat Asphyxia): A very fatal nervous affection resulting from exposure to extreme solar heat, and especially to the direct rays of the sun shining through a dry or highly electrical atmosphere. There are excessive thirst, faintness, cessation of perspiration, constipation, and paralysis of all the functions of the brain. Convulsions may be present or absent. In the former case the patient should be put into a tepid bath medicated with *Feb. 2.* Cold water should be poured into this, so as to reduce the temperature of the body to the normal point. In the latter case the neck and shoulders of the patient should be douched until the temperature is reduced below 104°. In both cases give *Feb. 1* lit. dil. alt. *Scrof. 1* in very frequent doses. Apply *Red* alt. *Yellow* El. to 2, 3, 18, 17, and forehead, also to soles of feet, and ointment of *Scrof. 5* alt *Canc. 5* to head.

Swallowing, Difficulty of: Treat like Laryngitis.

Swellings of Face: *Scrof. 1* first or lit. dil. alt. *Feb. 1.* Compress of *Scrof.* Ointment of *Scrof. 1* or *5*, or *Lin.* Applications of *Red* alt. *Yellow* El. to 3. 17, and masseter muscle.

Sycosis: An excrescence at the roots of the hair or beard, which in its fully developed state resembles the interior of a fig. At first there are small red patches which cause much irritation. This is followed by successive crops of pustules. *Scrof. 5* third dil. alt. *Ven.* second or third dil. *Scrof. 1* alt. *Canc. 5* lotion.

Syncope: See Fainting

Synovitis: Inflammation of the membrane which secretes the fluid by means of which the inner surface of joints are lubricated. *Ang. 2* alt. *Canc. 2*, and alt. *Scrof. 2* in lit. dil. *Ang. 2* and *Scrof. 1* ointment.

Syphilis: a repulsive disease which is developed in the system after a specific poison has been introduced into it through a mucous membrane or through any broken skin. The virus may be introduced through contact with a pipe, fork, spoon, &c., which has been used by a sufferer from the disease. It may be communicated by vaccination. Ordinarily, however, those who are affected by it have only themselves to blame for their affliction. Had they treated the sisters of others as they would have wished others to treat their own sisters, and had they remembered that the moral law points out the shoals on which man is in danger of wrecking his truest happiness, they would not have been doomed as they now are to suffer one of the most horrible of diseases. Within from 3 to 10 days after exposure to infection the syphilitic poison gives rise to an ulcer (chancre), which may be indurated, suppurative, ulcerative, or sloughing. Afterwards may follow chronic enlargement of one of the glands of the groin (bubo), mucous tubercles inside the cheeks, on the rectum, &c. ulcers of the tonsils and larynx, iritis, acute and chronic periostitis, and various other diseases of the bones and their coverings, intractable ulcerations of the nose, lips, &c. In treating the original ulcer give *Ang. 3* or *1*, litre or second dil. to check inflammation and congestion, and apply compress of *Ven.* to the ulcer four times a day. On the second day *Ven.*, litre dil., alt. with *Ang. 3*, and give 5 globs. *Canc. 5* night and morning. Sitz baths of *Canc.* 5 alt. *Ven.* Baths of *Canc. 5* and *Ven.* Should the ulcer not cicatrize give *Scrof. 1* in dil. instead of *Ang. 3* and apply compress of *Scrof.* 5 in alternation with those of *Ven.* In cases were bubo assumes the type of a phagedemic ulcer alt. *Ang. 3* with *Canc 1*, and use compresses of *Ang. 3* and *Canc. 5* with *Green* El., and apply *Red* alt. *Yellow* to corresponding nerves. In venereal orchitis give *Ang. 3*, third dil., alt. *Scrof. 1*, third dil. alt. *Ven.*, litre dil. When the infection has affected the whole constitution use the same remedies. Also baths of *Canc. 5* and occasional baths of *Ang. 3*, with *Red* alt. *Yellow* El. to 5, 18, 17. In hereditary syphilis *Scrof.* and *Canc.* are to be used rather than *Ven.* In all cases care must be taken to reduce the dose at once if any discomfort is produced. *Ven* is a very powerful remedy and must be used cautiously. If possible, in this, as in all other serious diseases, the patient should place himself under the care of a competent medical man who has studied the uses of the Mattei remedies.

Tape Worms : See Worms.

Taste, Loss of: This may be owing to change in the mucous membrane, nervous disturbances or disease of the nerves. *Scrof. 1* first dil. *Red* El. to 6, also in compresses to nape of neck and under the ears.

Teeth ; (1.) *Difficult Dentition :* This may be caused by scrofula or rickets; or it may result from improper feeding, want of sufficient fresh air, &c. Give *Scrof.* to the nurse; apply *Canc. 5* ointment to the infant's gums and *Red* alt. *Yellow* El. to the angles of jaws. If there are symptoms of brain irritation, a *little Ang. 2* ointment to spine, and *Feb. 2* to 24.

(2.) *Caries of :* Decay gradually penetrating towards the centre. This may result from want of cleanliness, the use of food which is either very hot or very cold, smoking, rickets, &c. Care should be taken to clean children's teeth regularly. *Canc. 1* second dil. Dry glob. of *Canc. 1.* Gargle of *Canc. 5, White* or *Blue* El. Compresses of *Green* El. *Canc. 5* ointment to nape of neck, and lotion of *Canc. 5* and *White* El. to cheek.

(3.) *Toothache:* This may result from inflammation of the tooth pulp, through exposure to a draught, digestive derangement, dental caries, impaction of the wisdom teeth, &c. 3 globs *Scrof. 1* dry on the tongue. Compresses of *White* or *Green* El. Gargle of *White* El. Applications *Red* El. if the pain is on the right side or of *Yellow* El. if on the left, to the external point of pain and to the gums, and of *White* El. to temples, side of nose, and behind the ears.

(4.) *Syphilitic Teeth :* The victims of inherent syphilis are liable to have dirty, grey, narrow-pointed teeth. There is a crescentic notch in the cutting edge of the superior permanent central incisor. Treatment as in Syphilis.

Tenesmus: Painful straining at stool. This is a characteristic symptom of Dysentery and of various local diseases. Treatment according to the cause; also enemata of *Scrof. Giap.* or *Canc. 1*, 20 globs. to tumbler of tepid water.

Testicles:

Cystic disease of. See Cysts.

Dropsy of. See Hydrocele.

Inflammation of the Testicles. See Orchitis.

Orchitis: Inflammation of the Testicles. See Orchitis.

Varicocele. See Varicocele.

Tetanus: An obscure disease. The nervous centres which control the voluntary muscles are abnormally irritated, and muscular spasms follow. Apply *Yellow* El. to the nerve centres affected. *Scrof. 1* second dil.; *Canc. 3* and *Lin.* baths.

Tetter: For Branny Tetter see Pityriasis; for Dry Tetter, see Psoriasis; for Soft Tetter, see Herpes.

Thread Worms: See Worms.

Throat, Sore: Simple inflammation of the mucous membrane at the back of the mouth, resulting from catarrh. *Feb. 1*, second dil., alt. *Scrof. 1*, second dil., or *Domfin. Feb. 2* ointment to 24. Compress of *Domfin*. Gargles of *Domfin* and *White* El. Inhalations of *Scrof. 1* or *5* are useful.

Clergyman's Sore Throat: Irritation, congestion, and subsequent relaxation of the lining membrane of the fauces and pharynx. The patient at first feels a desire to swallow; afterwards his voice becomes hoarse and the pharynx becomes painful. There is often much hawking. *Scrof. 1*, litre dil., alt. *Ang. 3*, second dil. 1 glob. *Domfin* hourly; *Red* alt. *Yellow* to 9, 13. Gargle of *Scrof. 1*, (4 globs.) *White* El. (4 drops) and a teaspoonful of glycerine to half-tumblerful of water. Gargles of *Blue* El. *Canc. 5* ointment to 6, 9, 13. Compress of *Canc. 5.*

Men who are liable to this affection should, if possible, wear beards. See also Laryngitis, Pharyngitis.

Throat Deafness: See Deafness.

Thrush (Aphthœ): small vesicles on the lining membrane of the mouth. There are also feverishness and pain on swallowing. Sometimes the eruption extends to the stomach and bowels. *Scrof. 1*, *Ang. 2*, or *Canc. 5* in second dil. Wash, with a hair pencil, the interior of the mouth with *Blue* El. and *Canc. 5*, 3 globules of the latter to a teaspoonful of Electricity.

Tic-Doulourex: Facial Neuralgia. For treatment see Neuralgia.

Tinea: See Sycosis.

Tongue, Cancer in: See Cancer.

Cracked or Fissured: arising from indigestion or irritation through decaying stumps of teeth. *Canc. 5*, litre dil. alt. *Scrof. 5*, litre or second dil. Gargles of *Canc. 5* alt. *White* El., or of *Scrof. 5* alt. *Red* El. *Red* alt. *Yellow* El. to 6, 9, 13.

Ulcer in: If syphilitic or cancerous, treat as in Syphilis or Cancer.

Tonsillitis: Inflammation of the tonsils. *Scrof. 1*, litre dil. Gargles of *Scrof.* alt. *Ang.* and *White* or *Blue* El.

Tonsils, Cancerous: Ointment of *Ang. 2* alt. *Lin.*

Toothache: See Teeth.

Trismus, Lockjaw: A symptom in tetanus. Apply *Yellow* alt. *Red* El. to cheek and 17, and if necessary, also to 18. Compress of *Canc. 5* and *White* El. to jaws. *Scrof. 1*, first dil.

Tubercular Meningitis: See Meningitis.

Tuberculosis: The production of tubercle. In the acute form of this disease the symptoms resemble those of typhoid. *Scrof. 1* alt. *Canc. 1* alt. all in second dil. *Canc. 5* ointment.

Tumours:

1. *Cancroid.* See Cancer.

2. *Cystic.* See Cysts. *Scrof. 1.* *White* El. compress.

3. *Fibroid:* Masses of fibrous tissue which may be hard or soft. Uterine Fibroid: *Ang. 3* third dil. alt. *Canc. 1* second dil., and *Red* El. compress; *Red* alt. *Yellow* El. to 5, 18. Baths of *Canc. 5* alt. *Scrof.* Injections of *Canc.*

5 alt. *Ang. 3.* If hæmorrhage sets in use third dil. of *Canc. 1*, and give one or two injections of *Ang. 3.*

4. *Osteomata :* Tumours composed of bone. *Canc. 4.*

5. *Scrofulous : Scrof.*; *Red* El. When suppuration commences, *Scrof.* alt. *Canc.*

6. *Sebaceous :* These are generally excised, but they may be treated with *Lin.* or *Canc. 5* ointment.

See also Condylomata, Hydrocele, Varicocele.

Typhoid and Typhus Fevers : See Fevers.

Ulcers : A breach of surface, with secretion of pus. Some ulcers heal readily. Others do not heal, either through defect, excess or peculiarity of action.

1. *Healthy ulcers* may be covered with compresses of *Scrof. 5* or *Canc.*, or of *White* or *Blue* El., (10 to 15 drops to a teaspoonful of water) covered with oiled silk. *Scrof. 1*, first or litre dil.

2. *Weak, Indolent or Chronic Ulcers* : Compress of *Canc. 5* alt. *Ang. 3. Scrof. 1*, litre or second dil. 1 glob. *Canc. 5* every 3 hours. 5 globs. *Scrof. 1* at meals twice daily.

3. *Irritable and Inflamed Ulcers* : *Scrof. 1*, second dil. alt. *Canc. 1*, second dil. Compress of *Green* El. and *Canc. 5.*

4. *Phagedæmic and Sloughing Ulcers* : Treat like Gangrene.

5. *Varicose Ulcers* : *Ang. 2*, second dil., or *Ang. 3*, second dil., alt. *Scrof. 1*, first dil. Compress of *Ang. 2* and *Blue* El. alt. compress *Scrof. 1.* If there is suppuration *Ang. 3* or *2*, second dil. alt. *Canc. 1*, first dil. Compress of *Canc. 5* alt. *Ang. 2.* This promotes suppuration at first, then gradually decreases it. When this happens

substitute *Canc. 2*, second dil., for *Canc.*, first dil. Afterwards use *Scrof.* to promote cicatrization. The leg should be supported with a Martin's bandage.

6. *Rodent Ulcers* : A tumour which begins as a pimple and, after a time, perhaps after some years, ulcerates and spreads. Its surface glistens and is uneven. A thin purulent discharge flows from it. *Feb. 1*. second dil., alt. *Canc. 1*, second or third dil. Compress of *Canc. 1* alt. *Canc. 5*. If there is any hæmorrhage give a few teaspoonfuls daily of *Ang. 3*, second dil. Compress and baths of *Canc. 5* alt. *Canc. 1* or *Lin.*

7. *Scorbutic Ulcers* : *Scrof. 1* alt. *Canc. 1, 2*, or *5*. 2 globules *Ang. 3* at dinner. *Red* alt. *Yellow* El. to 5, 18, 17. Baths *Canc. 5* alt. *Scrof.* 1, alt. *Ang. 3*.

8. *Bed Sores :* Compress of *Scrof. 5*, *Canc. 5*, and *Green* El. *Scrof. 1*, litre dil.

9. *Syphilitic Ulcer* : See Chancre, Bubo, Syphilis.

Uræmia : A nervous condition resulting from defective secretion of urine. In chronic cases there are listlessness, dimness of sight, drowsiness, torpor, and often convulsions and vomiting. In acute cases the patient may rapidly become comatose, or he may have one or several convulsive fits; or, again, he may be attacked both by convulsions and by coma. *Ang. 3* or *2* alt. *Scrof. 2* alt. *Canc. 5*. *Feb. 2* ointment to 24 and *Lin.* to lower part of spine.

Urethritis : Inflammation of the urethra. *Scrof.* alt. *Canc.* Sitz-baths of *Scrof. 1*.

Urethra, Stricture of the : This may be organic, inflammatory or spasmodic. When stricture has occurred, a scanty muco-purulent discharge takes place. Subsequently there is a frequent desire to pass water, and the size of the stream is very small. The patient may also suffer occasionally from retention of urine. *Scrof. 1* lit. dil. Compresses of *Scrof.*, *White* El., *Canc. 5*; injections of *Scrof. 1* or *Canc. 5*; *Red* alt. *Yellow* El. to 20, 22, 25; sitz-baths of *White* or *Red* El.

Urine: Albuminuria (Bright's Disease). At first, *Scrof. 1* first dil., with compresses of *Scrof. 1* or *Canc. 5* to the loins and *Red* El. to 20. If this fail, *Canc. 1* first dil. alt. *Scrof. 6* first dil.; 5 globs. *Scrof. 5* at meals; baths of *Canc. 5*, alt. *Scrof. 5* or *1*, alt. *Ang. 3*; baths *White* El.; *Red* alt. *Yellow* El. to 18, 17, 20, and spine. If there be any feverishness, *Feb. 1* second dil., and *Feb. 2* ointment must be added. Chills must be carefully avoided.

Dysuria: Difficulty in passing water. *Scrof. 1* lit. or second dil. alt. *Ang. 2* second dil.; 2 globs. *Scrof. 6* every four hours; *Red* alt. *Yellow* El. to 20 and spine; baths of *Canc. 5* alt. *Scrof.* alt. *Ang. 3*, and of *White* or *Red* El.; *Ang. 3* ointment to 20 and heart.

Hæmaturia: Bloody urine. *Ang. 3* second or third dil.; *Blue* El. to kidney region; compresses of *Ang. 3* to same part; baths of *Ang. 3*.

Incontinence of: *Scrof. 1* or *6* second dil.; *Canc. 1* second dil.; *Canc. 5* ointment and compresses to pubes; *Red* or *White* El. to 20 and 18; 1 glob. *Scrof. 5* dry every four hours; baths of *Canc. 5*.

Retention of: In children this may arise from worms. Treat as for worms, adding *White* El. compresses to 20 and apply *Red* and *Yellow* El. to 20. If the patient is of a sanguine temperament, *Ang. 2* second dil.; 1 glob. *Canc. 5* hourly; *Blue* El. to 20, 22, 25, 18, groins; baths of *Ang. 3* alt. *Lin.* If the patient is lymphatic, 1 glob. of

Scrof. 5 hourly; *Red* El. to 20, 22, 25, 18, groins; baths of *Lin.*

Sugar in: See Diabetes.

Urticaria: Nettle-rash. A form of Erythema (which see). It is sometimes caused through eating shell-fish or other irritant foods, by uterine irritation, scratching, bites, of insects, &c. It may be evanescent or persistent. The eruption consists of white prominences on the skin with a sensation as if one had been stung by a nettle. While the feverishness lasts, *Scrof. 1* alt. *Feb. 2*, second or third dil. *Scrof. 5* lotion over the rash. *Feb. 2* compress to 24. After the fever has gone, *Scrof. 1*, litre dil. 3 to 5 globs. *Scrof. 1* morning and evening. Tepid baths of *Scrof. 1.*

Uterus, Diseases of: See Womb.

Vaccination, Maladies consequent on. Advancing knowledge respecting disease germs has strenghtened the conviction, long felt by many, that Herbert Spencer was right in assuming that various diseases of the lymph and skin, even erysipelas and syphilis, may follow upon vaccination. And it is doubtful whether the evils of vaccination do not outweigh its benefits. To prevent development of any diseases which may follow it, *Scrof. 1*, second dil. Compress of *Scrof. 5*. Baths of *Lin.*

Varicocele: Dilatation and elongation of the veins of the spermatic cord. *Ang. 3* or *2* litre dil. alt. *Scrof.* litre dil. Compress of *Canc. 5* alt. *Ang. 3* and *Blue* El. Sitz-baths of *Ang. 3* and *Blue* El. alt. *Canc. 5*.

Varicose Veins: Dilatation and elongation of one or more veins, with hypertrophy of the coat. The veins may become tortuous, and varicose ulcers may be formed. *Ang. 3* or *2*. 3 globs. *Lin.* at meals. Compress of *Ang.*

2 or *3* alt. *Canc. 5*. Applications of *Blue* El. *Canc. 5* ointment and baths.

Phlebitis: Inflammation of the coats of a vein.

Venereal Disease: See Syphilis.

Vertigo: Swimming of the head: Dizziness: This may be caused by disorders of the eye, stomach, or brain. It may be a symptom of nervous exhaustion. It accompanies migraine and may occur in epilepsy. *Ang. 1*, third or second dil. 2 drops *Blue* El. *Ang. 2* compress to back of head. Friction of *Blue* El. to heart. If proceeding from the spleen *Feb. 1*, second dil. *Feb. 2* ointment to 24.

Vision, Defects of: See Eye.

Voice, Loss of: This may result from hysteria, paralysis of the adductor muscles, &c. *Scrof.* *Red* El. to 5, 12, 18 and 6. Gargles of *Ang. 2* and *Blue* El. *White* El., *Domfin*; Baths of *Canc. 5* alt. *Ang. 3*.

Vomiting: Expulsion of the contents of the stomach effected through excitement of the vomiting nerve-centre by irritation of certain afferent nerves which act upon it either directly or through the medium of the brain. The nerves which most easily produce vomiting are the nerves of the stomach, liver, kidney, bladder, uterus, ovaries, and especially the branches of the glosso-pharyngeal nerve to the root of the tongue, the soft palate, and the pharynx. At first 10 globs. *Scrof. 1* dry. Afterwards *Scrof. 1*, second dil. *White* El. to bottom of stomach. *Red* alt. *Yellow* to 5, 6, 18, 17. Same treatment in pregnancy. At Sea: See Sea-sickness. If persistent, resulting from liver disorder, *Feb. 1*, litre dil. *Feb. 2* ointment to 24. *Red* alt. *Yellow* El. to 6, 18. 5 globs. *Feb. 1* in the morning.

Vomiting of Blood: See Melæna.

Vulvitis: Inflammation of the vulva. *Scrof. 1* lit. Sitz-baths of *Scrof. 1* alt. *Scrof. 5.*

Warts: *Canc. 1* second dil. alt. *Scrof. 1*; *Canc. 5* ointment, compress or lotion.

Weakness, General: *Scrof. 1* lit. dil., 5 globs. at meals twice daily; *Red* El. to 18.

Wen: *Canc. 1* second dil. alt. *Ang. 3* second dil.; 1 glob. *Canc. 5* every two hours; compresses of *Canc. 5*; applications of *Red* alt. *Yellow* El. to base of gland and neighbouring nerves.

White Leg: See Phlegmasia Alba Dolens.

Whitlow: See Paronychia.

Whites: See Leucorrhœa.

Whooping Cough: See Hooping Cough.

Womb, *Colic of*: *Feb. 1* second dil.

Congestion of the: *Canc. 1*, 2 dry globs. every morning, *Lin. 1* second or third dil. alt. *Ang. 3* second dil.; 5 globs. *Scrof.* at meals; injections of *Canc. 5*; *White* El. to 20; baths of *Canc. 5* alt. *Ang. 3.*

Displacement: *Canc. 1* or *2* second dil.; injections of *Canc. 5.*

Falling of: *Canc. 2* second dil. alt. *Ang. 2* second dil.; *Red* alt. *Yellow* El. to 20; compresses and baths of *Canc. 5* alt. *Ang. 3* or *2*; compresses of *White* El.

Inflammatory diseases of: *Scrof. 1* lit. dil. alt. *Ang. 3* second dil. alt. *Canc. 1* second dil.; baths, unctions and compresses of *Canc. 5*; injections of *Canc. 1*; *White* El. to 20, 25.

Nervous affection of: See Hysteria.

Pains in: *Canc.* lit. or second dil.; sitz and whole-body baths of *Canc. 5*; *Canc. 5* compresses to abdomen.

Polypus of: *Canc. 2* second dil. or *Canc. 4* second dil. At meals, 4 globs. *Scrof. 1*, alternating this with *Ang. 1* second or third dil. if hæmorrhage sets in. Injections of *Canc. 2*, *Canc. 4*.

Spasms of: *Canc. 1* second dil. alt. *Scrof. 1* second dil.; or a dry globule dry every 20 minutes, lengthening the interval as soon as relieved. Compresses of *Canc. 5* and *White* El. to 20; baths of *Canc. 5* alt. *Ang. 3*.

Ulceration: *Canc. 1* second dil. alt. *Ang. 3* second dil. Injections of *Canc. 5*.

Worms: Over fifty parasites infest man's body. Thirty-five of these have their habitats within the frame. The commonest are thread-worms (oxyuris), round worms (ascaris lumbricoides), and tape-worms (tænia solium). The first give rise to local irritation, and frequent desire to go to stool, picking of the nose, and restless sleep. The second may cause distention of the abdomen, local itching, straining, nervous disturbances, grinding of teeth, dilated pupils, &c. The third may produce a sensation of weight or gnawing in the abdomen. In most worm cases the alimentary canal is in a disordered state, much slimy mucus is secreted in the lining of the intestines, the tongue is slimy, loss of flesh occurs, and the breath is disagreeable. The only sure proof of the presence of worms is the discovery of the parasites or of their ova. It must be remembered that in many cases worms are a cause of failure in the treatment of other diseases. *Ver.* lit. or second dil.; 2 dry globs. at meals; 2 to 5 dry globs. night and morning. Injections of *Ver. 2* and *Yellow* El.; *Ver. 2* ointment over abdomen. In some cases 5 to 10 drops of *Yellow* El. may also be taken fasting, in a dessert spoonful of water, two or three times a week. *Yellow* El., however, should be avoided by patients who suffer from hæmorrhage. Before commencing treatment for tape-worm it is well to give a dose of decoction of senna.

Wounds: If bleeding, after gently washing the wound, apply compress of *Ang. 3* and *Blue* El. Afterwards compress of *White* El. or *Green* El. If there is any suppuration or sloughing, apply compress of *Canc. 5* and give *Canc. 5* in litre dil. Should gangrene set in, give *Canc. 4*, litre dil. or *Canc. 10*, litre dil. alt. *Ang. 2*, litre dil., and apply compress of *Scrof. 5* alt. *Canc. 10*, alt. *White* or *Green* El. It may be noted that *Ang. 3* and *Blue* El. will stop bleeding; *Scrof.* will hasten cicatrization; *Canc.* should be used if there is suppuration.

Writer's Cramp: See Cramp.

Wry-neck, Torticollis: *Red* or *Green* El. to muscles of neck and to 17, 18, with *Scrof.*, first or litre dil. If there is fever give instead *Feb. 1*, second dil., and apply *Feb. 2* ointment to 24. Baths of *Canc. 5* or *Lin.*

Yellow Fever: See Fever.

Zona: See Shingles.

Principles of Electro-Homeopathy.

The efficiency and superiority of small doses of medicines in curing diseases, when applied according to the law of similars, is a fact that can no longer be disputed. A drug able to produce fever destroys it when introduced into the body in attenuated doses. Homeopathy, by applying this principle, has continually obtained remarkable results. Electro-Homeopathy is a new step in developing and perfecting Homeopathy. It excels Hahnemann's discovery in simplicity and reliability, its remedies also gaining more curative powers through the peculiar manner in which they are prepared. The word electro (or electric) is suggestive of the prompt action of the remedies and distinguishes them from the regular homeopathic ones. The discoverer of the new method is Count Cesare Mattei, of Italy, who starts, like Hahnemann and Rademacher, from the true principle that every disease is caused by vitiated fluids in the system, and that a cure can only be obtained if directed against those altered fluids, lymph and blood. Every disease is produced by the vitiated condition of the blood or lymph, or both. Whether the immediate cause be germs or noxious gases, etc., is of minor importance as far as the treatment is concerned, because the remedies act on the blood, lymph, or nerves and enable the organism to disengage itself from the morbid principles causing the abnormal condition. Consequently, there are three principal remedies, each including different potencies, a few auxiliary remedies, and the fluid electricities.

Electro-Homeopathy is a revolution in medicine. It is the medicine of the future, for many so-called incurable diseases can be radically cured; certainly not in the very last stages, but even then relief will be given and perhaps a cure obtained. That "there is no remedy for death" is certainly true, but there is no reason why man should succumb to so many diseases heretofore considered incurable.

The supposition that there is an amazing number of incurable diseases is quite inconsistent with the idea of an Almighty Providence, and is unworthy of that universal wisdom which has erected the tree of good by the side of the tree of evil, and which, in a word, has placed everything in the world that is necessary to salvation, be it in either a moral or physical sense.

The brute, guided by instinct, goes to browse on the herb that cures him; man has more than instinct: intelligence is the guide which should suffice to sustain his existence.

The cure must be a radical one, not allowing the disease to return after a short time. On the action of these remedies the organism recovers perceptibly; with the remedies penetrating the system, the general development and nutrition revive, the disease vanishes, the fluids are refreshed and renewed, the muscles strengthen, and the mind recovers its elasticity and activity.

Reflecting on these facts, established in inumerable cases, one must wonder why these remedies have not been discovered long ago.

Electro-Homeopathy teaches us a new kind of treatment by most effective remedies, to be applied internally, in the same way as Homeopathic remedies, as well as externally, thus producing much greater results than would be possible for Homeopathic remedies.

The action of the Electro-Homeopathic remedies proceeds in two principal directions, according to the disease resulting from either a vitiated condition of the blood or the lymph. Hence in every case the electro-homeopathic treatment takes for its base the constitution of the patient, being either lymphatic or angioitic (sanguineous).

The way of preparing the remedies is a complicated one, following the doctrine of the Spagyrics of the middle ages. The way of compounding the different remedies, i. e., the combining of the different series of plants into one remedy, which forms Count Mattei's discovery, remains his secret. The remedies are prepared under his own management, thus warranting their genuineness.

The remedies of the Spagyrics, so much renowned during the middle ages, contained the most effective ingredients of plants in a concentrated form, and required but a few drops to give the most satisfactory result.

By this method the power of every plant is entirely extracted; there is no other method of preparing remedies, either allopathic or homeopathic, to compare with this one. Selecting the elements according to the principles of Homeopathy redoubles their power. The prompt action of the vital fluid extracted from the plants is similar to that of the physical electricity. For this reason Count Mattei called it Vegetable Electricity.

Head-ache, tooth-ache, or neuralgia receive instantaneous relief from the application of the proper vegetable electricity; in the same way Green Electricity acts on cancerous wounds, on rheumatic and gouty pains, soothing the pain almost immediately.

There are no two constitutions alike. The dissimilarity of individuals varies infinitely according to age, sex, habits and the influence of their surroundings.

Hence we have the different forms and the complications of disease, though all arising from the same cause: vitiation of the lymph or of the blood.

In everything simplicity is the seat of truth. The new science has simplicity for its stamp and its demonstration, for every man can test the truth and the reality of its effects Trial and experiment would prove the truth of our theory to the medical profession, only too much disposed to condemn instead of giving a trial. There are, however, physicians who stick to the motto: Try everything and take the best. The true and the good work their way and the thousands of cures effected by the sufferers themselves, by clergymen and teachers, show better the nature of our method than all statements to the contrary made by jealous professionals.

The action of the remedies is a prompt one, not seldom instantaneous, a few grains of Antiscrofoloso taken dry on the tongue prevent or cure fainting or a stroke of paralysis; with the first tablespoonful of a solution of Anticanceroso the cramps of the womb quiet down or disappear; grave stinging pains and spasms surrender almost in every case to the fluid electricities.

The human body retains its form and the ability of the different organs to perform their functions by a continual change of its elements, which takes place from the moment of its inception.

By the incessant vital work the molecular elements of the organism are wasted and have to be replaced by new ones. Blood and lymph, the two fluids which may be considered the principal elements of the human body, supply the necessary matter.

Through the circulation the blood spreads itself throughout the organism, leaving everywhere new elements in its passage and carrying with it those already wasted in order to supply other parts of the body with them or to convert them into products of elimination.

Health is a normal state, resulting from a certain number of forces distributed through all the organs of the body according to a given law. From the brain to the finger's end, all has a part to fill for the support of life; everywhere is work and therefore consumption of force and transformation of matter. This is why the same matter cannot suffice indefinitely to support life.

The worn-out particles must be eliminated, leaving the body by the lungs in the shape of water, carbonic acid and so forth; by the kidneys and urine in the shape of water and other constituents of urine; by the skin as sweat, and by the bowels; to replace the waste and preserve equivalents the body takes food: (1) water for moderating the heat and helping to eliminate the worn-out particles; (2) carbonaceous food, like sugar, fat, farinaceous food, and (3) nitrogenous food, like meats.

While the transformations of matter take place normally, the frame is supplied with the elements necessary for its vital work and remains in a healthy condition.

The normal continuation of the vital functions, assimilation and elimination, constitutes perfect health, which is itself the result of the balance between the force wasted and the force renewed. Hence the elimination of exhausted matter represents the waste, whereas, the assimilation of food is the restitution. Perfect health is thus found subordinate to the physiological process of which we have spoken—that is to say, it is necessary that the atoms which pass from the food by assimilation into the tissues deposit there as much energy as the system has lost in the work of elimination.

The human body consists of numerous organs, derangements of which are more or less dangerous to life; every one of those organs, in fact the whole frame, hair and nails excepted, is fed by the blood, and in turn eliminate, through the blood and the lymph, their wasted products. Thus it is obvious that a derangement of the blood or lymph causes a derangement of the organs, and a diseased organ causes vitiated blood or lymph.

Health is subordinate, as we have said, to the normal transformation of matter; any derangement of it must be followed by some derangement of the vital work; that is to say, by some disease.

The lymph vessels form a net-work of small vessels, little tubes, similar to the smaller blood vessels, spreading through the whole system, permeating here and there different small glands, the so-called lymphatic glands; if inflamed and swollen from taking cold they will easily be observable in the back of the neck, on each side of the spine, etc., like a string of beads; after vaccination a swelling occurs of those in the arm-pit, and in certain diseases of those in the loins. These lymph vessels carry a white, milk-like fluid from the different organs to the *vena cava* (hollow vein), where this fluid mixes with blood and is transformed into blood, by means of oxygen, just before entering the heart.

Health depends on the normal conditions of blood and lymph, and every disease may be traced to some derangement of the blood or the lymph, or of both together; therefore there are two general series of remedies: those which act on the lymph, which are called Antiscrofoloso, and those which purify the blood, which are named Antiangioitico. By means of these remedies the constituent elements of all parts of the body are brought back to their normal condition. These elements, by the work of their gradual substitution in all parts of the body, cause the expulsion of disease germs wherever they may be found. Hence it results that in purifying the blood the action extends through the entire system, thus destroying disease. Hence, again, the reconstruction of wasted and partially destroyed tissues is no longer an impossibility. All diseases disappearing by using a certain remedy arise from the same source; that is to say, originate either from vitiated blood or lymph. Hence, it results that all diseases curable by Antiscrofoloso are caused by alterations of the lymph, whereas all diseases disappearing by the use of Antiangioitico will be traced to some alteration of the blood, and, finally, that all diseases requiring the proper use of both of these remedies result from a vitiated condition of both of these elements. It remains to say that the kind and the seat of a certain disease are insufficient indications for selecting the proper remedies; they can be used only as a means to ascertain whether the blood or the lymph, or both together, is vitiated. Every inflammation of the skin, for instance, may present itself in different forms; but to select the proper remedy it must be known whether it results from the diseased lymph or the diseased blood.

Hence a diagnosis is extremely easy; if the pulse, the arteries, the heart and the other symptoms indicate no defective state of the circulation it is only the lymph which is the cause of disease.

Electro-Homeopathy is not palliative like all other existing medical systems; it acts on the blood and the organism. To make this easily understood let us say: these remedies act on the sick in the same way as food does on the hungry. The more food the hungry will take the more the hunger will disappear.

In the same way the invalid will overcome his disease, using the proper remedies for the necessary length of time.

That a remedy used is the proper one is shown by the improvement following its use.

To sum up, the application of the remedies is easy. The vitiated lymph, produces a disease of the lymph, vitiated blood a disease of the blood. In cases of grave disease both blood and lymph are vitiated. Whether the blood or the lymph, or both together, is affected by impurities is understood from signs on the surface of the body. That knowledge is not difficult to obtain, the patient being the most able to give it, as experience goes to show. A sick man will never say: I am suffering from Leucoma, Sarcoma, Etmoplasma or Heteroplasma; but be says: I am suffering from Cancer. No sick man will say: I am suffering from congestion of the brain, or from deranged circulation, but he says: The blood is flowing to the head; I am afraid I will be struck by apoplexy," etc., etc.

Every disease, whatever its form may be, results from impurities of the blood or lymph, or from both together. If agents are discovered acting on the blood or the lymph, then the remedy is discovered.

The allopathic school of medicine admits that its remedies are palliatives; that is to say, they make disease disappear or cover it, but they do not cure in the real sense of the word.

If the facts are now well established that two general remedies and some auxiliary remedies destroy the cause of sickness, and that every disease arises from the lymph or the blood, how could it be possible for a man of common sense not to cure himself? Is it possible not to distinguish between an eczema and an irregular palpitation of the heart? Can it be possible to mistake varicose veins for tetter? But even if such a misunderstanding should occur, no other inconvenience can result from it than the failure to effect a cure. Thus the remedy itself gives us a warning that we are wrong and have to substitute the other one of the two general remedies. It can not be toc often repeated, that every disease arises from the blood or the lymph. This is therapeutics in a nutshell.

Every one of these remedies acts on the system in accordance with the Homeopathic principle of similarity: "*Similia similibus curantur.*" Every one of those remedies develops its healing power only when it meets with a certain well defined, so to say, congenial pathological condition; in every other case no effect will be produced; if the remedy is appropriate to the disease, but the dose too large, an aggravation of the symptoms will follow, but will disappear after administering several doses of the proper attenuation of the same remedy.

The Homeopathic probings of the action of drugs on the living, necessary with the Hahnemannian school, are not admissible with these remedies, because they are not poisonous.

The fundamental axiom of Homeopathy, by which only that remedy can cure a disease entirely which produces similar symptoms in a healthy person, is to be modified in Electro - Homeopathy, that any Electro-Homeopathic remedy is properly selected if liable to produce in a larger dose an aggravation of the symptoms.

Besides the internal remedies we have in Electro-Homeopathy the five fluids for external use, called Electricities.

The name Electro-Homeopathy is derived from the fluids called electric on account of their quick action. There are green, blue, yellow, red and white electricities, so called from the color of the bottles they were formerly dispensed in.

The specific action of the electricities is on the nerves, aiding the internal cure in a remarkable way.

After knowing what the constitution of the patient is, the lymphatic individual is to be given Scrofoloso, the angioitic Angioitico and in addition Canceroso, if the case is a grave one. Special indications for giving Canceroso are glandular and cancerous troubles and wounds.

If the patient is of a mixed constitution he needs Scrofoloso and Angioitico alternately; when there is a doubt whether the patient is lymphatic or angioitic, use Scrofoloso 1 or Scrofoloso 5, because most people are scrofulous; or treat the disease as combined, alternating Scrofoloso with Angioitico. To these principal remedies the specifics are to be added sometimes; thus in fevers the Febbrifughos, in affections of the lungs and the bronchiæ the proper Pettorale, in cases of syphilis Venereo, and in cases of worms Vermifugho are to be added alternately.

The remedies of the different series numbered one, having the widest sphere of action, the treatment of every case is to begin with No. 1, unless there are special indications justifying the application of some other number.

The ordinary dose for an internal remedy is one grain dissolved in three-quarters of a water-glass of water. This is called the first dilution and is taken by tablespoonfuls; in aggravated cases a teaspoonful is to be taken every 15 minutes. If the remedy be well selected an improvement will be observed after taking the first few spoonfuls in acute cases, otherwise after three to four days; in grave chronic cases after six to eight days. If the remedy produces aggravation the remedy is right, but the dose is too strong. The second dilution must then be taken. Take a teaspoonful of the first dilution, put into three quarters of a glass of water, this is the second dilution. Should even that one prove too strong, or have no effect at all, the third dilution is to be taken and prepared in a like manner as the second.

If no change occurs within the time given above and after diminishing the dose, either the remedy was wrong or the destruction of the organs has reached such an advanced stage as to make a cure impossible.

As a general rule, the graver the case the weaker the dose must be and the more frequently administered, a teaspoonful every 5 to 10 minutes. The effect of the remedy in the dilutions is instantaneous, but not lasting, therefore the doses must be repeated in rapid succession to obtain a cure.

.Experience shows that cold climates require stronger doses than warm climates.

Improvement is indicated by diminished symptoms, by increased sweating, expectorations, thick urine, by an abcess forming, or diarrhea; the body, stimulated by the remedies, striving to get rid of its bad fluids through various channels. Sometimes improvement seems to stop, sometimes a relapse occurs. One must not be troubled about the one or the other, for these remedies often subdue the most aggravated and apparently incurable cases, the most complicated cases resisting every other treatment; necessitating, however, a treatment that will require time.

The old school of medicine describes several hundred forms of cancer, not one of which it can cure. What difference can it make to the patient to know exactly whether his cancer is of a fungoid or gelatinous nature, whether it is an epethiloma, a scirrhus, a sarcoma, a leucoma, a carcinoma, a neoplasm or a heteroplasm, or any other such sentence to a painful death. One would really think that we were pretending (as the Chinese do) to scare away the cancer with horrible sounding words. It is strange that, when our civilization is advancing with such rapid strides, every one has been attending to details, and no one to what should be our principal aim and object, the art of healing; that our scientific men should have submitted to such prodigious toil and study, in order to describe and name a disease which they do not know how to subdue and cure.

Allopathy has several hundred kinds of cancers with frightful names; in Electro-Homeopathy all is reduced to one – cancer—that is to say, one great morbid principle in the blood, which shows itself chiefly in the form of malignant tumors, which keep growing larger and larger, and never stop till they have developed into an open sore. The knife of the Allopath removes the product, the result of the corrupted blood; but the blood itself cannot change, so the cancer grows again after the operation. On the contrary, Electro-Homeopathy has the power of changing the corrupted blood, of changing the constitution; and this is why, instead of 1,100 fearful names, Electro-Homeopathy knows but one, that of cancer, which it can cure more or less quickly, according as the corruption of the blood is more or less advanced. But even where death results, Electro-Homeopathy always shows its beneficial action by the amelioration of all the principal symptoms, such as more or less stony hardness, and the shooting pains in cases where the tumor is closed; and the deeply fixed and rooted nature in the case of open sores, the black or yellow color, the raised and hardened edges, the discharge which may affect any tint, from the color of water to that of ink; the pains, the fetid smell, &c., &c. And by the influence of Anticanceroso, and Antiangioitico 3, &c., you will see a gradual change takes place in all the above characteristic symptoms, even in the more serious cases. What you will obtain in one and all of the cases treated, is the cessation of pain.

In cholera, as in cancer, the same farce performed by the old school of medicine goes on. One theory ascribes its origin to bacilli; another to microbes; another argues that you must not call them microbes, but macrobes. Some say it is caused by little organisms, others by organisms armed with stings. Some say it is caused by flies; some say that it is adhesive and contagious; some think that it is to be found in the rarified air of the mountains; others in the heavy air of the valleys. Alas, for science! It is the remedy that we want.

In this Guide some points are repeated intentionally, in order to impress the memory of the reader. As stated below:

"Every alteration of either one of the two liquids, blood or lymph, must with the accompanying nervous influences necessarily lead to an alteration of the normal state of the individual and produce an abnormal or pathological state. Taking this theory as a base, it is easy to understand that the composition of the remedies, called Electro-homeopathic, on account of their efficacious and often instantaneous action, should embrace a group of simple medicinal principles which, in virtue of their nature and mode of action upon the whole of our body and the various parts which compose it, would be able to meet the demands of sundry morbid elements which in altering the normal state of the blood and the lymph constitute all diseases, that is to say, the hostile causes which are opposed to the free exercise of our organic functions."

All the medicines of Count Mattei have been extracted from innocuous plants and no harm is ever produced by taking them in a healthy state of the body or by mistaking one for another. These medicines produce on the body a mild, sometimes an almost instantaneous, but more generally gradual action, in such a manner that the effects are perceived only after the administration of two or three doses, or after some time.

They purify the blood and free the system from morbiferous and extraneous matters by increasing the perspiration, evacuations, expectorations and deposits in the urine. Very often also a mild diarrhoea, free from all pain, sets in and thus removes the morbid principles that were the cause of the sufferings.

As the greater number of diseases are due to vitiation of the lymph, the treatment in almost all cases should be commenced with Scrof. 1. Experience, says Count Mattei, proves that the 2nd dilution is generally the best.

In very *Violent Diseases* take a tea-spoonful every quarter of an hour, or even every five minutes.

If this treatment has no good result, or if the result is not complete, take A. in the same manner as S 1, either alone or in alternation with S 1, that is, take one hour a spoonful (or a tea-spoonful every quarter of an hour) of A. and the other of S.

If even by this treatment no complete cure is brought about it shows that the disease is far advanced and deep rooted, and requires a more powerful remedy. Take therefore C 1 in the same manner as S., either alone or in alternation with A. or S., according as you think that A. or S has done you more good.

In case of diseases of the chest use P.; in case of fevers F.; in case of worms Ver.; and in case of syphilis Ven.

Use the specifics whenever indicated, but generally only after having tried A 3, S 1, C 1; for it is only rarely when A 3, S 1, C 1 have not produced a complete cure, that they are required.

The dose must be diminished according to the violence or gravity of the disease, and in this case the number of spoonfuls taken must be increased.

A chronic disease will necessitate the use of the second or third dilution, while acute, or sudden cases will require the first dilution or from 10 to 15 dry globules; as, for instance, cases of fainting, hysteria, epilepsy, and other nervous disorders. The treatment is then continued by a dilution of the remedy which had been administered dry.

As a rule, the doses are the same for children; for nursing infants the remedy may be given to the mother.

Patients should be particularly warned not to increase the dose, taking two, three or more globules instead of one, in order to get cured the more speedily. This will not do. They will either not get cured at all, delay the cure, or what is worse, bring about a relapse by this foolish action.

People are to be cautioned against a sudden interruption in taking the remedies, especially the Cancerosos, because of the possibility of a relapse. The best way to do is to continue the treatment for some length of time after the disappearance of all symptoms: in light cases for half the time of the original treatment; in graver ones for the same time. In cases of cancer and organic troubles, it is advisable to never stop taking the remedies; it is then sufficient to take the grains dry or with the meals.

Count Cæsar Mattei's

Electro-Homeopathic Medicines.

According to the theory of Count Mattei all the diseases the human frame is subject to, arise from the vitiation or derangement of the lymph and blood, and more particularly from the former. To restore them to their normal state, and the body to health, it requires medicines which have the power to destroy the morbific poisons permeating the blood.

These correctives or restoratives the Count has discovered.

THE ANTISCROFOLOSOS.

Antiscrofolosos cure all diseases arising from the vitiation of the lymph, which they restore to their normal condition and thus do away with all the ailments its vitiated state gave rise to. Vitiation of the lymph is indicated by swelling of the Glands, Derangement of the Stomach, Tumors, Boils, Eruptions and other Skin Diseases.

Antiscrofoloso is therefore generally required in Anæmia, Asthma, Colic, Calculi, Diabetes, Diarrhœa, Dropsy; Flow of Saliva, Tears, Bile, Urine, Pus, White Matter, etc.; Flatulence; Incontinence or Rentention of Urine; Indigestion, Leprosy; Loss of Appetite, Taste, Smell, Hearing, Voice; Lumbago, Obesity, Sting or Bites of animals; Inflammation of the Kidneys, Bladder, Eyes, Ears, etc.; Sadness; Stone, Skin Diseases of all kinds, Sciatica, Ulcers.

Of all the medicines of Count Mattei S 1 and S 5 have perhaps the most powerful and the widest sphere of action as they have to be employed in almost 90 out of a 100 cases of sickness.

It may also be used as a preventative, as it purifies and preserves the body from bilious and scrofulous principles and promotes good appetite and digestion. There are 7 numbers of Scrofoloso:

1. ***Scrofoloso 1*** (abbreviated Scrof. 1, or S 1). It has the widest sphere of action of all the remedies. It is the remedy for Scrofula, for most cutaneous diseases, etc.; effective in every case, because of spora occurring in every organism, especially for eruptions—gout—itch—scabies—scurf—rachitis—caries—consumption—elephant-

iasis—morbid fatness—atrophy—inflammation of the eyes —deafness— convulsions (if originating from the lymph) — asthma — ischias — cataract — polypus — mania — staphyloma.— Catarrhal angina—diphtheria—granular sore throat—chronic inflammation of the tonsils—gastritis—gastric ailments of women—sea sickness—indigestion — vomiting—loss of appetite — gastralgia — ascites with general dropsy dependent on organic abdominal disease—diarrhœa—obstinate constipation—marasmus—asthma—glandular swellings—disorders of the urinary and generative system—kidney disease—diabetes—coxalgia—articular rheumatism—hysteria — epilepsy—fainting—boils—carbuncles—all kinds of skin disorders — erysipelas — ulcers — fistulas—whitlow—all kinds of eruptive fevers—megrin—neuralgia in the head —disorders of the eye—ear—and nose—chronic coryza —all disorders dependent upon anæmia.

Taken daily with a beverage, during meals, it induces sleep, appetite, strength, and is a preventive of disease and infection.

2. ***Scrofoloso 2.*** (Abbreviated Scrof. 1, or S 1.) also called Scrofoloso Nuovo.

Gastric and rheumatic fevers (with Febrifugo 1) — loss of hair—megrim—hysteric neuralgia—nervous and chronic dyspepsia—goitre—glandular swellings in the neck - catarrhal cough—croup — hoarseness— chronic venereal disorder, (with venereo)—paralysis of the hands—sciatica—cramp in the legs.

Scrofoloso 2 must not be taken for an attenuation of Scrofoloso 1; quite to the contrary, it is a different remedy, composed of special constituents.

This remark applies to all other members of a certain series, having something common in regard to their principal action on the lymph or the blood, but well distinguished in regard to their specific action.

3. ***Scrofoloso 3*** (Scrof 3, S. 3). Also known as Scrofoloso Doppio.—Facial eruptions—herpes—gastralgia—hernia—glandular swellings —weakness in the

generative system—arthritic nodes—debility—infantile convulsions, epilepsy.

5. ***Scrofoloso 5*** (Scrof. 5, S. 5), acting on the blood also; is mostly used for skin and blood diseases. —All skin disorders—eczema—lupus—red and swollen eyelids—glandular enlargement—chronic laryngitis with ulceration (with Canceroso)—granular throat—chronic indigestion from the retrocession of skin disease— chronic constipation — abdominal phthisis — hæmorrhoids — chronic rheumatism - sciatica — vomiting—diarrhœa—colic—frost-bite—chronic coryza —renal calculi—gravel—incontinence of urine.

6. ***Scrofoloso 6*** (Scrof 6, S. 6). Specific for scrofulous wounds. — Specially adapted to diseases of the bladder and kidneys—diabetes—rheumatic affections in the joints of the hands and feet—muscular weakness.

Giappone—or Scrofoloso Giappone (abbreviated, Scrof. Giap. or G.). This is the anti-choleraic remedy, and is specific in most disorders of the digestive apparatus—as in vomiting—diarrhœa—dysentery—cholerine and cholera, and the fever connected with these diseases.

Linfatico. (Linf. or L.) *Linfatico* is an intermediate remedy between the *Angioitico* and *Scrofoloso* groups, and is employed in unctions, frictions, compresses, baths, etc. Internally it is used in vertigo with nausea — gastric debility— headache— toothache— dental fistula—blind and fluent hæmorrhoids—glandular enlargement and induration—gastric and other fevers (with Febrifugo)—kidney diseases—premature menstruation with colic before or after—generative debility— lymphatic complaints of children. The daily use of this remedy, in doses of 4 to 10 globules, strengthens the constitution in mixed or nervous temperaments. It is especially effective against pains (from wounds or ulcers), glandular ailments, etc.

Marina. (Mar., or M.) For all diseases of the eyes, as staphyloma, cataract and inflammation of the eyes, ophthalmia and all mucous membrane disorders.

THE ANTIANGIOITICOS.

Angioiticos cure all disorders arising from a vitiated state of the blood, irregular circulation, etc. It modifies, corrects and regulates the blood, restores it to a healthy state and eliminates the morbific poisons which impeded its circulation. Vitiation of the Blood is indicated by Palpitation of the Heart, Violent Beating of the Arteries, Vertigo, Rush of Blood to the Head; Loss of Blood from the Nose, Stomach, Anus, Urinary Organs, etc.; Coldness of the Extremities, Corns, Warts, Varices.

Antiangioitico is therefore generally to be used in Apoplexy; Swelling, Inflammation and Beating of the Arteries; Heart Diseases, Dropsy of the Spine: Pericarde, Chest, Kidneys, Loss of Sight, Congestion, Chlorosis, Deranged Menses,Constipation,Dysentery, Paralysis, etc.

1. ***Angioitico 1*** (Ang.1, or A 1) has a special action in all disorders of bilious and nervous constitutions—inflammatory fevers—typhoid fever (with Febbrifugo)—neuralgias — cerebral congestion — congestive headache — encephalitis — meningitis —inflamed eyelids — acute and phelgmonous sore throats—quinsy—nervous asthma—pleurisy — convulsive cough — spitting of blood—acute inflammations of the generative organs—metrorrhagia and too copious menstruation—metritis—cystitis—menstrual colic—rheumatic and gouty inflammations with swelling. A specific for paralysis (if caused by defective circulation).

2. ***Angioitico 2*** (Ang. 2, A 2) for all disorders of the circulation, of the heart, veins, arteries—congestions—varices — aneurisms — hæmorrhoids — hysteric disorders arising from deficient vitality in the uterine system — articular rheumatism — epilepsy — jaundice (with

Febbrifugo)—inflamed ulcers—metritis—metrorrhagia—sciatica—enteritis—pneumonia—pleurisy—hœmoptysis. A specific for piles or hæmorrhoids.

3. ***Angioitico 3*** (Ang. 3, A 3). The most effective in cases of alteration of the blood; also for nervous affections.—Chronic skin disease—nettle rash (with Scrofoloso 5) — congestions — sunstroke — hæmorrhagic apoplexy — paralysis — gastritis — enteritis — constipation with sanguine temperament — ulceration and cancer of the stomach (with Canceroso), asthma—quinsy —chronic laringitis—acute and chronic pneumonia—acute bronchitis—uterine cancer, etc.

THE CANCEROSOS.

The remedies of this group, have a special action against all diseases which reach such a point that they resist the action of the *Scrofoloso* medicines.

1. ***Canceroso 1*** (Canc.1, C1). Remedy for diseases of the lymph and for cancer. The treatment by the Cancerosos has to begin with this remedy. It acts especially on scirrhus, cancers, white swelling, glands, polypi, inflammation of the ovaries and all troubles of the womb, falling, bending and pains of it—leucorrhœa. A single grain in a glass of water hastens and alleviates delivery. Canceroso 1 is also used in the following disorders: Scirrhus and other cancerous conditions of the breast—cancer of the stomach, tongue, the shin, the nose, lips, uterus, etc.;—white swellings—spasms—fainting spells—and hysteric attacks — disorders of pregnancy — uterine cramp—leucorrhœa — dropsy — ascites — wasting disease in children—inflammation of the rectum—induration of the liver (also Febbrifugo)—phthisical symptoms—granular laryngitis—ulcerative or granular throat—diphtheria—all kinds of lung diseases—scurvy —mumps —spinal disease —cerebral congestion—acute and chronic gastritis—typhoid fevers (with Febbrifugo)—diabetes—disorders of the generative system in both sexes.

2. ***Canceroso 2.*** Canceroso Nuovo (Canc. 2, C 2). It is a specific for glands (tonsils) and dropsy, and is used in uterine disorders which do not yield to Canceroso 1, especially when attended with hypochondriasis.

3. ***Canceroso 3,*** This remedy is also called Canceroso Doppio (Canc. 3, C 3). Specific for cancer of the stomach and (lymphatic) fibroides, etc., and may be recommended in the following cases: White or inflammatory swelling of the knee, paralysis of the joints, of the hands and feet, resulting from rheumatism, or sprain, or dislocation—cancerous ulcers—cancer on the lips, breast, etc.

4. ***Canceroso 4*** (Canc. 4, C 4). Especially in cancerous caries and inflammation of the bones, etc.

5. ***Canceroso 5*** (Canc. 5, C 5), the ladies' remedy. It is for internal and especially for external use in cases of cancerous ulcers, diseases of women, miscarriage, leucorrhœa, change of life, ovarian troubles and every disease pertaining to the female organs. It is one of the most powerful of all, and the one most generally used in baths. With Pettorale it is specific in pulmonary excavations, in scirrhus, induration, cancer in all external parts, all kinds of ulcers--chronic eruptions—scurvy and scrofula—diphtheria—phthisis—laryngitis—megrim—ascites—dysmenorrhœa—leucorrhœa—deafness--lachrymal fistula—cataract and chronic eye disease—amaurosis—dyspepsia—acidity--gastralgia—and all acute disorders of the stomach.

6. ***Canceroso 6*** (Canc. 6, C 6). An excellent cancer specific, is a remedy indicated in gastric and bilious disorders--infantile cholera—metrorrhagia—in weak and unhealthy women—cystisis—kidney disease—uterine tumors—purulent ear discharges, etc., etc.

10. ***Canceroso 10*** (Canc. 10, C 10). For internal and external use in cancer, it combines the action of all the rest of the canceroso medicines.

Canceroso T. B. (Canc. T. B., or T. B.) This remedy is a specific for all urinary troubles, bladder and kidney diseases. Inflammation of the urethra, stone in the bladder, pus in the urine, bloody urine, deposits and sediments in urine, retention of urine, etc.

Dom Fin. (D. F.) This is comparatively a new remedy. It is, especially in the second dilution, a specific for diphtheria, and all throat troubles: Quinsy, croup, sore throat, consumption of throat, hoarsenes, membranous croup. It is in diphtheria that it has gained such renown.

Lord. (L.) *Lord* is useful in umbilical hernia, and in many cases of cancer. It belongs essentially to the cancerous group, and may be often advantageously used as an intercurrent remedy in these diseases.

THE FEBBRIFUGOS.

1. ***Febbrifugo 1*** (Febr. 1, F. 1). Specific in all kinds of fever—intermittent—periodic of all types—remittent—neuralgia, etc. Febbrifugo also cures all disorders of the liver and kidneys—acute and chronic spleen diseases — hypochondriasis.

Febbrifugo 2 (Febr. 2, F. 2). Very efficient in all cases of fevers and affections of an intermittent type, and diseases of the liver and the spleen, is always associated with Febbrifugo 1 in the diseases for which that remedy is required; it is administered in unctions and compresses to the abdomen and hypochondria. Sometimes it is used internally in obstinate cases which resist the action of Febbrifugo 1.

THE PETTORALES.

Usually taken in the second dilution, the same as the other remedies, that is to say,

in serious cases, alternately with the Pettorales, take Canceroso, or Angioitico 3, according to complications, one dose every 10 to 15 minutes.

At meals one may take a few globules of Scrofoloso Giappone, as an extra remedy when taking Pettorales.

Bronchial patients troubled with thick greenish expectoration can be cured with Pettorale No. 1.

The thick clotted yellowish and gray expectorations indicate sores on the lungs, which can be cured with Pettorale No. 2.

Tuberculous patients can be cured with Pettorale Nos. 1 and 2.

Catarrhous patients have an abundant whitish and very liquid expectoration, and can be cured with the Pettorale Nos. 3 and 4, which are specially suitable for such cases.

1. ***Pettorale 1*** (Pet. 1, P. 1). Specific for diseases of the air-tubes, of the lungs or bronchiæ and of the chest, coughing, etc., also in whooping cough—croup—loss of voice—chronic obstruction in the lungs—rheumatic laryngitis—tracheal and pulmonary phthisis—pneumonia—chronic hepatisation of the lungs, ædema of the lungs, etc.

2. ***Pettorale 2*** (Pet. 2, P. 2), is specially indicated in pulmonary cavities(with Canceroso), pneumonia with hæmorrhage, and pulmonary emphysema. Also used externally in washes, salves, baths, inhalations, gargles, etc., indicated in catarrh of the bronchial tubes —chronic pulmonary catarrh, and all kinds of cough.

3. ***Pettorale 3*** is more suited to children than the other forms of Pettorale.

4. ***Pettorale 4*** (Pet. 4, or P. 4). For old chronic cases in which everything has been tried without avail.—In night sweats, last stages of bronchitis, consumption, change of voice, cheesy expectoration, etc.

VENEREO.

Antivenereo (Ven.), subdues every kind and stage of syphilis, being also its preventive. For all forms of venereous (syphilitic) diseases, if not degenerated into cancerous affections, then Canceroso also is indicated. As a preventive take one grain every half hour. Venereo is to be used for syphilis in all its forms and stages.

THE VERMIFUGHO.

Vermifugho 1 (Verm. 1). There are two Vermifughos, each of them efficient in removing all kinds of worms and sufferings therefrom, the small thread-worm, the long round-worm, the tape-worm, etc. The proper dose is the 2nd attenuation; should it prove inefficient, take from 5 to 40 grains in a glass of water.

Vermifugho 2 (V.2), as unction on the abdomen, groins and the flanks.

If yellow electricity is taken, 15 drops before breakfast, it is a powerful remedy for worms.

Anti Mal de Mer (Mal de Mer), (Ma. d. M.) A preventive and cure for sea-sickness and similar stomach troubles, especially with lymphatic persons. As a preventive for sea-sickness, take 2 grains every 1 to 2 hours.

Aqua Per la Pelle (Aqua Perl). Is for the skin and complexion. It is used externally for baths or washes. A teaspoonful to a pint of water. It purifies the skin, removes freckles, moles, rough skin, pimples, and makes the skin smooth and velvety. It is also used locally for sore and weak eyes.

FLUIDS WITH ELECTRIC QUALITIES.

Red Electricity (Elec. red, or El. r.)—having positive action.

Yellow Electricity (Elec. yell., or El. y.)—having negative action.

White Electricity (Elec. wht., or El. w.)—having a mixed action; is always beneficial.

Blue Electricity (Elec. bl., or El. bl.)—positive, especially adapted to angioitic and asthmatic persons.

Green Electricity (Elec. gr., or El. gr.)—negative, for cancerous wounds and rheumatism of the joints.

DIRECTIONS FOR USING THE REMEDIES.

Every treatment with the Antiscrofoloso has to begin by using No. 1, and with the Antiangioitico by using No. 3. As shown by experience these numbers are the most efficient in almost every case.

If, after taking these numbers, there is no improvement, then either the remedy or the dose is not appropriate, and another number is to be taken, instead of Antiscrofoloso 1 the Antiscrofoloso 2, etc., and so on.

If a remedy selected is not appropriate to the ailment no other inconvenience will be felt than a failure to cure. It is advisable to begin every treatment by Antiscrofoloso 1, because psora, as Hahnemann says, plays its part in every disease.

The action of the remedies is often instantaneous, as is shown in fainting, colic, drunkenness, threatening paralysis, etc. These affections disappear as soon as the proper remedy has been applied.

ABBREVIATIONS.

Abbreviations of the names of the different remedies are made by using the initial capital letter of the name and adding the number; for instance: Antiscrofoloso or Scrofoloso by S; Antiscrofoloso 5 by S 5; Antiangioitico 2 by A 2; Febbrifugo 1 by F 1; Vermifugho by Verm.; Antivenereo by Ven ; electric red—by el. r.

THE SERIES OF REMEDIES.

Every remedy, however efficient it may prove, does not act in the same way on every individual; hence it becomes necessary to prepare remedies of similar action in conformity with the individual requirements. For instance, if Scrofoloso 1 should prove insufficient, take Scrofoloso 2, 3, 5 or 6, etc.

How to apply these Remedies.

All globules for internal use may be applied externally as well, in the form of compresses, unctions, in baths, for gargles and inhalation.

DOSES FOR INTERNAL USE.

All the remedies may be used internally in three different ways.

In solutions, i. e. one grain dissolved in water. There are three such solutions.

1. The first glass, or the first solution, will be had by dissolving a single grain or powder in a common sized glass, three-quarters filled with water. This is to be taken by tablespoonfuls or by sipping. Usually a spoonful every hour, in aggravated cases every fifteen minutes.

2. The second solution, or dilution, will be had by pouring a tablespoonful of the first solution in a glass three quarters full of water. This solution, as well as the third one, is to be taken in teaspoonful doses.

3. In a like way the third solution is prepared from the second.

Workingmen and others not liking these solutions may use the pills. These pills are to be had at the agency, 330 La Salle Ave., Chicago. Price per ounce, or about 100 pills, 25 cents. One pill being equal to a teaspoonful of the respective solution. This way of taking the remedies is more convenient and equally efficient.

Or dry, i. e. from eight to ten times during the day, one grain on the tongue. Or ten to twelve grains are taken in a beverage, or with the meals.

We have observed how colic and dysentery were cured and threatening paralysis averted by giving the patient a solution of one grain of Scrofoloso 1 in a table-spoonful of water every three minutes.

In grave cases from forty to fifty grains must be given in a glass of water. Dr. Cricca in Smyrna and M. Schmid in the Hotel Rosa saved patients suffering from the most malignant fevers, declared hopeless, by giving forty grains of Febbrifugo 1 and forty drops of white or blue electricity.

Much depends upon the observation and sagacity of the person directing the treatment.

Dr. Pusheck very often uses the remedies in powders because of the great exactness possible in determining the dose of the remedy, thus preventing patients from altering doses by carelessness or other causes.

It is always to be remembered that the failure of a remedy to improve is caused either by the dose being wrong or the remedy being improperly selected.

With children the second solution is to be used. Sometimes the solutions do not agree with the patient; then the grains are to be taken dry.

EXTERNAL APPLICATIONS.

For a *full bath* (be it cold, lukewarm or hct) for a man one hundred grains, for a woman from sixty to eighty grains are to be used. The grains may be previously dissolved in a small quantity of hot water, and poured in the water just before entering the bath.

For a *local bath* of the arms, the legs, etc., from 20 to 30 grains are taken. The temperature of the water can be fixed at liberty.

Compresses. 20 to 30 grains are dissolved in a glass of water, to which a few drops of the respective electricity may be added. Compresses are to be removed as soon as dry, and renewed from three to four times a day at least.

Gargles. Dissolve from 20 to 50 grains in a glass of water.

Salves or Unctions. Fifteen grains are dissolved in a few drops of water and then well mixed with a tablespoonful of lard, olive oil, glycerine or vaseline. These unctions to be applied from four to five times daily. The most efficient and strongest unctions are those prepared by the agency: 330 La Salle Ave., Chicago. They may be kept for years.

Inhalations, Injections and Clysters. They should be prepared as prescribed for compresses; for inhalation the solution must be heated and then inhaled by means of some inhaling apparatus; for injections by means of a syringe.

Suppositories. This is another means of applying the remedies; they excel by cleanliness and effectiveness.

The *Vaginal Suppositories*, prepared from Canceroso and Green Electricity are an excellent remedy for all diseases of women, are a substitute for injections, and are much liked for good results, simplicity, and cleanliness. These suppositories are especially effective in cases of inflammation of the womb, irregular menses, ulcers, and suppurations of every kind, sterility and other diseases of the organ, for leucorrhœa, and in cases of insufficient and painful flowing, etc. Canceroso is also to be taken internally, having met with success in almost every case. Price 75 cents per dozen, 40 cents per half a dozen.

Before applying the suppository, oil it with a little lard or salve. The proper time is at bed-time; the suppositories will dissolve in from 1 to 5 hours by the natural heat of the body, the fluid condition giving the remedy an opportunity of acting directly on the involved parts.

Hemorrhoidal Suppositories. There is nothing like these suppositories for curing piles; they are used in the same way as the other suppositories and prepared from the powerful blood remedies: Blue Electricity and Angioitico 2. Specific against piles, golden vein, etc.

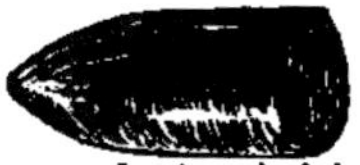

They relieve at once the stinging pains of piles, and by using them for some length of time piles will be entirely cured; Angioitico 2 must be taken internally. At bed-time and after every discharge of the bowels the anus is to be washed with cold water. Price per dozen 50 cents.

Compresses and unctions are to be renewed as often as the condition requires.

For baths, unctions, and compresses the electricities may also be used. For a full bath a tablespoonful, and for compresses and unctions a few drops are sufficient. — When there is no improvement after taking a certain remedy, another one is to be substituted; that is to say, for one of the Antiscrofoloso one of the Antiangioitico is to be substituted, or the red or the yellow or the blue electricity is to be applied.

ALTERNATING THE REMEDIES.

A patient obliged to take different remedies, say three, must take them alternately. He may choose to take one the first day, the other one the second, the last one the third day, or prefer using each of them for one-third of one day. He may take them alternately every hour, using the second solution. The action of the remedies being often electric, instantaneous, a remedy taken 5 minutes after the application of another one will interfere in no way with the action of the first one, its effect being already obtained. The instantaneous action of the remedies will be observed in pains; a woman suffering from spasms of the womb will usually perceive the pain to disappear after taking a few teaspoonsful of the first solution of Canceroso 1.

When using different remedies, the one most active in subdueing the disease under treatment must be given more frequently. For instance: Take the most efficient remedy in second solution in small doses, often repeated, all day long; give the remedies of less importance in a beverage during meals. The most important remedy for the time being is one which relieves the acute symptoms and not the one which destroys the actual cause.

Suppose we had to deal with a stroke of syphilitic apoplexy; then the Angioitico is to be applied first to relieve apoplexy; then the cause of the trouble will be cured by giving dissolved grains of Antivenereo during meals. After overcoming the main trouble, treatment is to be continued with Antivenereo alone.

ELECTRICITIES OR FLUID REMEDIES.

Red, Yellow, Green, White and Blue Electricity.

The most characteristic feature of Electro-Homeopathy are the five electricities with a specific action on the great nerve-centers, regulating the vital work. Through the medium of the nerves the electricities exercise a powerful influence on the blood and the lymph, rendering, if properly applied, an excellent means of aiding the internal treatment; in light affections and in pains even a cure will be effected by simply applying the electricities externally.

When applied where the nerves are nearest to the skin (for the right points of application see the drawings in rear), they will remove or at least soothe the pain; when pain is caused by vitiated blood or lymph the electricities may be used to advantage, but to effect a perfect cure the internal treatment is indispensable.

1. *The Red Electricity* with electric qualities (commonly called Red Electricity) has a positive action. It principally suits lymphatic organisms; it is applied in diseases of the stomach and the abdomen against neuralgic pains and sciatica, and in all cases where the body is in a negative electric condition.

If applied in the super-orbital and sub-orbital region it strengthens the eye-sight.

2. *The Yellow Electricity* with electric qualities (commonly called Yellow Electricity) has a negative action. It acts when neither of the others take effect. It also counteracts the red, and therefore neutralizes the too powerful effects of the red. It is especially useful where there is an excess of vital power. It is also specific for worms. Alternating the red with the yellow is of great advantage in convalescence.

3. *The White Electricity* with electric qualities (commonly called White Electricity) is neutral. It is especially used for affections of the head and diseases of the abdomen. Its action is always beneficial.

4. ***The Blue Electricity*** with electric qualities (commonly called Blue Electricity) has a positive action and acts on the veins. It is used for varicose veins, hemorrhages and all diseases of the blood. In cases of apoplexy it acts most powerfully if used internally; as much as fifty drops for one dose. Blue Electricity is indicated for sanguine or angioitic persons.

5. ***The Green Electricity*** with electric qualities (commonly called Green Electricity) is negative. Its pre-eminent action is on wounds, hastening cicatrization, also on pains of the joints. In all cancerous affections its effect is excellent.

The electricities are generally applied like a cupping glass. A small bottle with a wide opening is applied to the skin, where the nerves are nearest, and on the painful points of the muscles.

Yellow electricity is a good remedy for worms. Take a drop on a lump of sugar before breakfast; the number of drops may be gradually increased to ten. Green electricity is always used for compresses.

If the position of the patient prevents the cupping method of applying the electricities then pour a few drops on a piece of cotton and place it on the given points. A camel-hair brush may be used for the same purpose.

The application of the remedies should last from five to ten minutes, and is to be repeated frequently. Sometimes short and frequent applications act the best.

The question arises: Which electricity must be used to relieve pain or remove cramps, the positive or the negative?

Experience has shown and continues to show that both positive and negative electricity remove pain Health is the natural condition, and disease a disturbance thereof.

Well, which electricity is needed to restore the neutral condition?

Experience teaches us the fact that the positive electricity is useful in most cases, and therefore the red electricity is to be first applied, because of the prevalent negative condition of the body. If no effect is produced then take the yellow electricity.

If pain is not removed by the red electricity or by the yellow, the blue is brought into action. For in that case the pain results from an alteration of the circulation of the blood.

White electricity is appliable in all kinds of headache, tooth-ache, neuralgia of the face, etc. For pains of the joints apply the green.

The yellow electricity has an electric action on the tendons also. Every pain will be removed by one or the other of the electricities, unless there is a grave alteration of the blood or the lymph, in which case no help can be expected without internal treatment. Rubbing in of salve of Scrofoloso 1, Linfatico or Lord, or Canceroso 5, acts also as a pain-killer.

The internal remedy, subduing a swelling or a painful nerve, removes the trouble without any application of electricity, though it will take a longer time.

If the patient is decidedly angioitic, neither the red nor the yellow electricity is to be used but the angioitic or blue electricity.

It often happens that pain jumps from one part to another after applying the electricities; applications are then to be continued and the pain pursued from spot to spot until it is removed. A great remedy for pains of every kind is a bath of Scrofoloso 3.

For internal use commence with one drop of electricity in a tablespoonful of water and increase day by day to ten drops or even more, according to the effects. One way to take electricity is in two daily doses of ten drops each, mornings and evenings. If two doses show no effect, a third one of 10 drops is to be taken at noon.

If red electricity should have been applied to sufferers from cramps, to hysteric or plethoric persons, as sometimes happens by mistake, give the patient about ten grains of Scrofoloso 1.

In all cases continue the application of that electricity which has given the best results.

GENERAL RULES.

Electro-Homeopathy combats the causes of disease, not alone its results.

1. If a disease is not well defined, Scrofoloso 1 is the proper remedy in most cases, as the psoric condition prevails among all. If Scrofoloso 1 prove unsatisfactory, Angioitico is to be taken. This remedy will of necessity produce satisfactory results for the simple reason that the cause of any disease not seated in the lymph must be in the blood. Should Angioitico fail also, it is obvious that both the blood and the lymph are vitiated, and Anticanceroso, or, rather, Scrofoloso 3 has to come into action. These two remedies give excellent results in such complicated cases.

2. If any remedy not appropriate to the case should be applied, it can not do any harm, it will simply have no effect at all. This result is an indication of the necessity of using either a different remedy or a different dose.

3. The constitution of the different individuals and the remedies appropriate to them are understood from the following signs: Angioitic or sanguineous persons suffer from palpitation of the heart, vertigo, congestion, varicose veins, hemorrhages, cold extremities, etc., moreover, they have not much appetite, an irregular digestion, and often they are troubled with constipation caused by a sluggish circulation. For such persons the Angioiticos are the remedies.

4. If the patient has none of these symptoms, he is necessarily lymphatic, and the Scrofolosos and Cancerosos are his remedies.

5. Sometimes, rather frequently, a mixed condition exists; that is to say the condition is lymphatic and angioitic together. For such patients the Scrofolosos *and* the

Angioiticos are the proper remedies to be applied alternately. The angioitic symptoms in such cases are few and not well defined.

6. These patients must be treated with Scrofoloso *and* Angioitico; but according to the lymphatic or the angioitic condition prevailing, either Scrofoloso or Angioitico must have the preference.

7. There is no strict diet to be observed during treatment. Pure water aids the action of the remedies. As to diet, no restrictions need be observed. In grave cases a milk-diet is of great importance in connection with the remedies. Avoid sour or highly seasoned food.

8. Menstruation is no reason for discontinuing the treatment, the remedies giving greater satisfaction during that period than otherwise.

9. During pregnancy ladies may use the remedies without hesitation. One grain Canceroso 1 put in a glass of water removes the uneasiness during and hastens delivery.

10. It is of importance to remember that the effect of a certain remedy is the same whether it be applied internally or externally; by using it internally and externally at the same time, the effect is doubled and the recovery hastened.

11. If a remedy has no effect, it proves that:

a) The diagnosis was wrong, hence the remedy not properly selected, or

b) The dose was wrong, necessitating an attenuation of the dose, or

c) The disease has reached the latest stage, and is therefore incurable.

12. There are persons who may be helped by very small doses, and others who require very large doses both internally and externally. Whether the dose is to be attenuated or strengthened for a certain person remains for him to decide who directs the treatment.

A report in the "Moniteur" says: A person suffering from a malignant fever, and declared beyond all hope ten days ago, was cured after lying in a stupor for 24 hours with 40 grains Febbrifugo in water and 50 drops white electricity.

13. If a certain disease shows signs of disappearing through the action of some remedy the dose of that remedy has to be increased, because these remedies act according to the laws of similars. Therefore, if the disease is grave and serious, the dose is to be attenuated. In very critical cases a dose of 40 grains even may be given.

14. The treatment once commenced must not be interrupted while the disease exists, as it would expose the patient to relapses. To avoid this it is sufficient to take the grains dry at meals.

15. It should be well remembered that a certain remedy which was a success in one case will not prove a panacea in every case. For that reason not only a single remedy but a whole series of remedies should be at hand.

16. The treatment is to be continued for such length of time as is required. Not only the symptoms, but the cause must be removed. Hence the treatment must be continued for some time, even though the disappearing of the symptoms seems to warrant a cure. But then the remedies need not to be taken with such strict regularity; taking them during meals in a beverage is sufficient. This rule of continuing the use of the remedies after an apparent cure applies especially to grave cases.

REVIEW AND CONCLUSION.

Any and every disease, of whatever form it may be' even the most aggravated case, is the result of the vitiation of the blood or the lymph.

Electro-Homeopathy possesses two series of radical remedies: one for the blood, the other for the lymph. The effect of the remedies is the same, whether they be used internally or externally.

The Electro-Homeopathic Mattei remedies are made in small white globules, or pills, or grains. These three terms having practically the same meaning when referring to these medicines. The remedies are manufactured in this shape and are not sugar pills, simply moistened or saturated with some medicine, as ordinary Homeopathic remedies are. They are made and imported in this form. They dissolve much harder than Homeopathic sugar pills. The Electricities are a clear liquid,—in appearance like water.

Every remedy may be applied in three different ways, viz:

1. *Internally:* 1 grain in a glass of water or dry, one grain every hour.

2. *In grains:* 12 to 15 in a day; or from 6 to 10 grains mixed with a beverage during or after meals.

3. *Externally:* A full bath of 60–100 grains; gargles, injections or compresses prepared from a solution of 20 grains in a glass with water, and salves, 15 grains to a tablespoonful of olive oil or lard.

The electricities, though not apt to cure the blood, aid the power of the internal remedies by influencing the nerves.

Extraordinary results will be obtained from giving the remedies in rapid succession, say every three minutes.

A full bath of Linfatico will prove most beneficial in every disease.—A single grain of Scrofoloso 1 acts wonderfully in fainting fits, colic, drunkenness and sea-sickness, if taken dry on the tongue.

In desperate cases strong doses are the rule, from 40 to 50 grains in a glass of water, or from 40 to 50 drops white or blue electricity. Persevering pains, paralytic strokes, and malignant fevers are subdued by taking 100 drops white or blue electricity.

The blue electricity stops bleeding and cicatrizes even injured arteries. Applications to the back of the neck often meet with great success, acting on the nerves centering in the small brain and influencing the whole body.

The diagnosis in Electro-Homeopathy is very easy. If one is suffering from palpitation of the heart, dizziness, varicose veins, congestion, constipation, piles, cold feet, tingling in the hands or feet, the Angioiticos are the appropriate and efficient remedies. If those symptoms are missing there ought to be no hesitation in using the lymphatic remedies.

There are still other cases requiring both the Angioiticos and the Scrofolosos. This is always the case in serious diseases.

If a remedy is not properly selected no effect at all will follow. The remedies are harmless; 100, 1,000, even 10,000 grains of any of them given to a dog or kitten will prove it.

The diet is unrestricted; in grave cases acid drinks, lemonade, and other sour food preparations must be avoided.

Pains of the womb, pregnancy and troubles during confinement are alleviated in a wonderful way by Canceroso, and so are the many diseases of the womb.

In the same ratio as the disease disappears, the doses should be increased and the remedies given in each of the three different ways mentioned above.

To practice Electro-Homeopathy it is necessary to be conversant with the preceding principles and rules.

INDEX.